THE
G-CONNECTION

THE G-CONNECTION

◆

HARNESS GRAVITY AND REVERSE AGING

Dr. Joan Vernikos

with Robin S. Hosie

Foreword by astronaut and senator
John Glenn

iUniverse, Inc.
New York Lincoln Shanghai

THE G-CONNECTION
HARNESS GRAVITY AND REVERSE AGING

iUniverse, Inc.

For information address:
iUniverse, Inc.
2021 Pine Lake Road, Suite 100
Lincoln, NE 68512
www.iuniverse.com

ISBN: 0-595-32931-4 (pbk)
ISBN: 0-595-66710-4 (cloth)

Printed in the United States of America

Contents

Foreword

Look around and notice how the number of older Americans is growing. By 2050, the number of those over eighty-five is projected to increase by 600%; this will have all manner of social, economic, and medical consequences. My experience both in space and on the Senate's Special Committee on Aging convinced me we should capitalize on what we learn from astronauts in space to help our ever-increasing elderly population on Earth enjoy productive, healthy lives. This timely and comprehensive book by Joan Vernikos explains lessons learned from space in readable, understandable, and intuitively appealing terms. It gives practical recommendations on how we can best take charge of our health and maintain our independence.

I first met Joan Vernikos on June 18, 1996, when visiting NASA Administrator Dan Goldin. Also with me was John Elsold, the attending physician to Congress. We were discussing the relationship between space travel and the aging process, following on a well-received speech Goldin had delivered to the American Association for Retired Persons (AARP). I had already read widely on the subject and talked with NASA doctors, but I was curious to meet the author of *Parallel Processes: The Study of Human Adaptation to Space Helps Us Understand Aging*, which had grabbed my attention.

It was apparent that Joan Vernikos, director of life sciences at NASA, and I thought alike regarding the similarities between the physiological changes brought about by space travel and those associated with the aging process. More particularly, how could we best take advantage of the countermeasures we had learned to use for astronauts and apply them to treat the normal health problems among the elderly on Earth? On September 3, I had the opportunity to debate the matter in the Senate.

I already had the full backing of the National Institute on Aging. Joan Vernikos had developed an excellent working relationship with the National Institutes of Health and was now of considerable help in persuading them of the scientific merit of having a seventy-seven-year-old fly in space again. Yes, I had wanted to go back into space, but the main reason was to do research and acquire new information. The door to that research has now undoubtedly been opened.

The STS-95 Discovery flight resulted in a barrage of publicity, which focused people's minds positively on the aging process. Hardly a day goes by without an article in the papers or the expounding of new theories. Joan Vernikos pioneered the research method of putting healthy men and women in continuous head-down bed rest in order to study, on the ground, how the human body adapts to space flight. She brings to this book her particular expertise in such subjects as hormones and the stress response. Her intricate knowledge of these fields and her lifetime involvement with NASA make her ideally qualified to write this book for the lay reader with an inquiring mind. Best of all, the sections on "What you can do about it" make this a very practical book, utilizing the very best of both earth and space-based medicine for your benefit.

John Glenn
Former senator (D-OH) and astronaut

Introduction

My many years of research with NASA involved understanding the effects of space travel on astronauts. The ultimate goal was to find ways to protect them from any adverse effects. It soon became clear to me that astronauts, almost without exception young, fit, highly trained, and hand chosen, return from space missions feeling old beyond their years. Neither I nor any of my colleagues had any doubt that there was a link between space travel and aging—but what exactly was the nature of that link?

After turning the problem over in my mind for months, the answer dawned on me one day in July 1980. It was an answer in the form of a question. Could the link be gravity or rather the lack of its use here on Earth? In space, there is essentially no gravity. As we on Earth grow older we tend to give in to gravity. We sit down a lot more than we used to. We do not stand up as often or as energetically as before. We move about and exercise a lot less. We have invented clever ways of doing less physical work, with the invention of motor cars, self-propelling grass mowers, and household devices that require minimal effort. We even spend more time in bed reading than when we were younger. All these habits reduce the extent to which we use gravity, which has its maximum influence on our bodies when we are upright. As a result, we allow gravity to drag us down.

In order to test my theory I used methods on the ground that simulated the removal of gravity. The best of these reduced the gravity load by asking healthy volunteers to stay in bed from four to eighty-four days so we could study their physiological and psychological responses. It was this research, originally designed to help us develop countermeasures for astronauts, that convinced me that gravity, the force under which all life on Earth has evolved, is our body's friend and not its foe.

More importantly, it seemed to me that the countermeasure treatments we were testing in astronauts and our bed-rest volunteers could also be applied in order to delay, prevent, or even reverse many of the symptoms we commonly associate with old age.

We cannot escape growing older in years. But we can, with a positive approach to life, the right diet, activities, and exercises that capitalize on the gravity around us, stay young, healthy, and independent as long as we live.

Various non-technical audiences became increasingly interested in hearing more about this subject. At the end of my talks, many asked me, "Where can I find out more about this?" I knew of no reference work I could recommend.

This book is in response to that and other questions. It aims to put in plain language a multitude of research discoveries from space that may help us understand how we must constantly use gravity to improve the quality of our lives. By making your use of gravity a daily habit, like brushing your teeth, you will remain healthy and active here on Earth for as long as you live.

1

Do Astronauts Grow Older in Space?

○ ○

The advantage of living is not measured by length, but by use; some men have lived long and have lived little; attend to it while you are in it. It lies in your will, not in the number of years.

—*Michel de Montaigne (1553–1592), Essays*

We all grow up with preconceptions and make assumptions about the way things are. Then someone finds a new way of looking at the world and our myths are shattered. The Earth is not flat. Girls are just as good at math as boys. It is now possible for humans to leave Earth in their flying machines. A person with a broken spine will walk again someday soon, maybe not quite like you and me but unaided nonetheless. Another assumption that just about everybody shares is that advancing years bring about irreversible changes in body and mind, changes that signal an end to independence and the joy of living. However, it does not have to be so. And the evidence comes from a most unlikely source: space.

The Ultimate Challenge

They were stirring times, those early years when humans set out to conquer space. The Russians astounded the world when, in October 1957, they launched *Sputnik I*, the first man-made satellite to girdle Earth. This triumph was followed by another, even more spectacular. On April 12, 1961, Soviet cosmonaut Yuri Gagarin, in *Vostok I*, became the first human to be blasted into space. During a flight that lasted just over 108 minutes, he orbited Earth. There were parades, medals, cheering crowds, and broad smiles all around Moscow! In Washington, there was consternation. For this was the era of the Cold War, and a rocket powerful enough to launch a man into space could easily be modified to carry a more sinister payload, a nuclear warhead. America had to catch up and fast. The Space Race was on.

In May 1961, President John F. Kennedy challenged the country: "I believe this nation should commit itself to achieving the goal, before this decade is out, of landing a man on the moon and returning him safely to Earth." NASA, the National Aeronautics and Space Administration, which had come into being in 1958, delivered a swift and dramatic response. On February 22, 1962, John Glenn stepped aboard a Mercury capsule, which he named *Friendship 7*, to become the first U.S. astronaut to orbit the earth. I was at Ohio State University at the time, teaching pharmacology to medical students. Caught up in the sheer excitement of space, I knew instinctively where I wanted to be. By 1964 I had joined NASA.

As daring as President Kennedy's vision was, it was achieved with five months to spare. On July 21, 1969, former test pilot Neil Armstrong, commander of the *Apollo 11* mission, became the first man to set foot on the Moon. America had done far more than merely catch up.

Many new technologies were developed as a result of the Space Race: bar codes, quartz watches, ball pens that can write upside down, under water, and even on glass, communication satellites, computers, imaging techniques, cordless tools, a scratch-and-glare-reducing coating for sunglasses, a non-stick surface now used for frying pans, and so on. But we did not go into space to invent the non-stick frying pan. We went there because it was the ultimate challenge. And though these by-products have proven useful, they are eclipsed by another spin-off from the Space Race, one that is of vital importance to every man, woman, and child living on Earth. Research whose main purpose was to help American astronauts conquer space has led to a fuller understanding of how our bodies work. It led to a discovery that will certainly help people on Earth stay healthy and energetic throughout life, reversing and delaying many of the problems we usually associate with aging.

Gravity: The Common Link

Gravity is the force that keeps us rooted to Earth. It keeps the stars in their courses and the planets in their orbits. The gravitational pull of the Moon, nearly 240,000 miles away (384,000 km) from Earth, causes the regular swellings and retreats of the tides.

Into Space—at 25,000 mph

Gravity is measured in units known as "Gs," and the force that normally operates on Earth is designated as 1G. For a rocket to break free from Earth's gravitational field, it has to reach a speed of more than 25,000 mph (40,000 km/h). Achieving this from a standing start calls for a tremendous burst of acceleration, which increases the compression forces on astronauts to 5G or even 6G. Even though astronauts lie on their backs during launch to reduce the full impact of this hypergravity, it puts an immense strain on their bodies. This is one reason why they need to be in peak physical condition.

On Earth, the load of gravity on an individual can be increased by rapidly spinning the person on a wheel-like apparatus, called a centrifuge. In 1795, Erasmus Darwin, a physician and the grandfather of Charles Darwin, proposed using centrifugation to reduce fever, slow down the heart rate, and induce sleep! In the nineteenth century, centrifuges were used in Europe to treat the mentally ill. These earlier attempts did not survive the test of time. However, I believe hypergravity by centrifugation has other potential medical applications, which should become more apparent in the course of this book.

Centrifuges designed to carry humans can create a force as high as 20G, though no human can tolerate that level of force. Russian studies found most humans exposed to hypergravity in a rotating room could tolerate no more than 6G for several days, but they could live for longer periods at 2.0G. Fighter pilots may experience short bursts of 6 to 10G pulling in the head-to-toe direction, but only for a few seconds. At present, hypergravity is exploited mainly by amusement parks, in roller coasters and other fun rides. It pins thrill-seekers to their seats even when they are traveling upside down, with the floor above their feet. Near the other extreme, the pull of gravity on the Moon, which has a diameter only a quarter the size of Earth's, is as low as 0.165G. This is one-sixth of Earth's G. You could easily jump ten times higher on the Moon than you can down here.

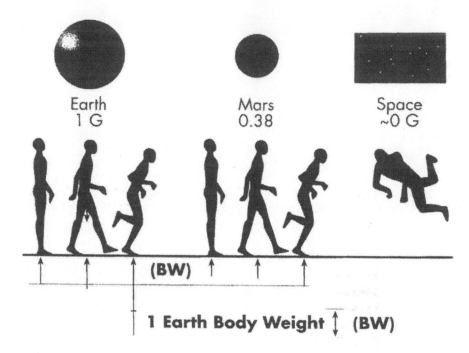

External forces on the body are a function of Gravity (G) and are amplified by activity. Mars has about one-third the gravity of Earth, and the Moon only one-sixth. Walking, running and jumping, amplify this force on the body. (By permission from J. Vernikos, "Human Physiology in Space," Bioessays 18:1029–1037,1996).

In 1666, so the story goes, Isaac Newton watched an apple falling from a tree, as millions had done before him. The difference was that Newton wondered about what *caused* the apple to fall. This led him to develop the laws of gravity and motion, which helped us understand the movements of the planets and made it possible for humans to explore the vastness of the cosmos.

My Personal Quest

My fascination with space was selfish. As a scientist, I knew the only way to find out how we are affected by something in the world we live in was to take that something away then observe how the body reacts. When scientists wanted to know how light affected humans, they studied what happened to them if they lived in darkness. To understand what role Earth's gravity had upon us, we had to go into space. At last it was possible to do that. But the primary objective of my research was to provide the knowledge and tools to make sure astronauts could live and work in space.

Well, you may say, what is so special about gravity? Everyone surely knows we live in gravity. We are surrounded by it. Aren't we all taught in school about Earth's rotation around the Sun and Newton's falling apple? Most of us are aware that what we weigh has something to do with gravity; a few, who aspire to a firm body by exercising with weights, perhaps realize they owe their benefits to it as well. And yet many of us are unaware of how gravity affects the way we look, feel, and function. The Space Race made it possible for the first time to explore the subject. The answers led to an astonishing insight for those of us living down here on Earth, one that established the fascinating link between gravity and aging well.

What Spaceflight Does to the Body

Nothing could be more unnatural for those of us who live on this beautiful blue planet than to step beyond gravity's reach. Every organ and function of the human body, indeed of every living creature, has evolved, developed, and taken shape under the burden imposed by gravity. The way we use this force determines how strong we will be in our prime, how well we function throughout life, and how far our skin will sag and muscles waste as we grow older. It is small wonder that traveling in space, where the pull of gravity is practically reduced to zero, can have a damaging effect on an astronaut's body. However, many of the consequences predicted by the National Academy of Sciences' experts did not happen. Astronauts can swallow in space, and their eyes do not fall out.

As long ago as 1961 and 1962, Soviet cosmonauts Titov and Nikolayev, who were the first to stay in space longer than twenty-four hours, had trouble maintaining their blood pressure when standing upon their return to Earth. Later, as flights grew much longer, this problem was so serious that cosmonauts had to be carried away from the landing site in reclining chairs.

Disturbed regulation of blood pressure turned out to be only one of a number of symptoms. Astronauts who took part in the Gemini and Apollo missions of the 1960s showed signs of reduced aerobic capacity and were losing calcium from their bones. A kind of anemia, caused by a reduction in the number of red blood cells, was diagnosed in astronauts returning from Skylab missions in the early 1970s. We now know that all the muscles, but especially those that support posture, will atrophy during spaceflight. Similar changes happen to the bones of the legs and lower spine, which lose strength and can become brittle. The digestive system is affected in a number of ways. The motility of the gut is reduced, so that it becomes sluggish. The body is less able to absorb calcium from the intestines.

The immune system is depressed, astronauts become more sensitive to heat and cold, and they often have difficulty getting a good night's sleep.

When astronauts return to Earth, their eyesight is not as sharp as it was. They find it hard to keep their balance, typically standing with their feet wide apart and walking with their legs further apart than usual. After long flights, they tend to shuffle and find it difficult to get around corners without running into walls.

As in Space, so on Earth

If you were asked what condition you would associate with the array of symptoms just listed, space travel would not be the first thing that came to mind. It is more likely that you would think of some of the old people you know. For the very same bodily changes experienced in an accelerated form by the astronauts are what we have come to expect, down here on Earth, from a process that is spread out over a lifetime, commonly known as aging. In 1984, I wrote a pamphlet pointing out these similarities.

I was not alone in my conclusions. In the mid-1980s, John Glenn, now a U.S. senator (D-OH), was chairman of the Senate Committee on Aging. As the committee heard testimony describing the various ills afflicting the elderly, it struck him that he had come across some of these ills in a different setting. Glenn was convinced that the high number of symptoms common to both spaceflight and aging was more than just coincidence. Ten years later, when I was NASA's director of life sciences in Washington, D.C., I well remember going by our public affairs office's TV set one day and glancing at a discussion on the Senate floor. Glenn was urging his colleagues to support Space Station while waving over his head a pamphlet on the parallels between aging and the effects of spaceflight. My pamphlet! I could hardly believe my eyes.

Glenn later used his influence to encourage the National Institute on Aging and NASA to work together on this subject. The rest is history. John Glenn's return to space at the age of seventy-seven—his nine-day flight on *STS-95* in October 1998—did more, by its very boldness, to increase public awareness of what space research could contribute to the cause of healthy aging than any scientist or scientific report could ever have done.

Do You Age Faster in Space?

I am often asked if I believe that astronauts grow old faster in space. The answer to this is a resounding "No." The changes that happen to astronauts in space are appropriate for life in space. They are only abnormal compared to their condition before going into space. It is when the spacecraft begins to re-enter Earth's atmosphere and comes in for landing that these changes become serious problems.

All astronauts, whatever their age, show signs of physical deterioration as they experience gravity again. But with a little time, these changes can be reversed. Astronauts recover fairly quickly after their flights. Follow-up observations and annual physicals have shown that the recovery is permanent. This mysteriously telescoped *space aging* is a problem that lasts only as long as they are learning to cope with gravity once more, after living, even for a comparatively short time, in this highly unnatural environment—a world without gravity.

That is clear enough. But what, then, is the exact connection between spaceflight, gravity, and aging? The answer came from the research we were doing on the ground to find ways of supporting the health of our astronauts in space.

Lying in Bed for the Sake of Astronauts

Human beings are more affected by gravity than most other animals because of our erect posture. The maximum effects of gravity occur when we are upright and its force is pulling in the head-to-toe direction. All you have to do to reduce its impact is to sit down—or, more effectively, lie down. When you do so, gravity is only pulling across the width or depth of your body, not along its length. This simple fact is of enormous importance in explaining the relationship between spaceflight and aging.

The Space Race provided both the motivation and the resources to discover ways of safeguarding the health of our astronauts. All we needed was a research method, a way of coming as close as possible on Earth to reproducing the "zero gravity" effects of flight in space (and, of course, sufficient volunteers willing to subject themselves to our research). The number of human beings who can be sent into space is limited, and they have more than enough to do without being subjected to constant tests and experiments. To date, the number of both astronauts and cosmonauts who have flown is only around 400. We needed to study far larger numbers if we were to build up a databank big enough to point to solid conclusions regarding the links between gravity and health and to develop ways of preventing the unpleasant bodily changes suffered by astronauts in space.

Epidemic That Led to an Inspiration

First, the method. We tried several, including one that seemed, for a time, to show some promise: immersing a volunteer's entire body in warm water, with only the head above the surface. This certainly reduces the pull of gravity on the mass of the body, but it has major drawbacks. After twelve hours of soaking, the body becomes macerated. Breathing becomes difficult, and the sensory deprivation involved can cause psychological problems. The immersion method was thus abandoned as impractical.

Instead, we turned to a more manageable way of mimicking the effects of going into space—putting people to bed and asking them to stay there for days, weeks, even months. This method came from an inspired medical observation. Until the Salk vaccine became available in the 1950s, every summer seemed to bring an epidemic of the viral infection poliomyelitis somewhere in the world. Franklin D. Roosevelt, in his early thirties, was the best-known victim of this viral infection, which results in crippling paralysis of the muscles and serious bone loss.

In the early 1940s Don Whedon, at the National Institutes of Health, in Maryland, questioned whether the bone loss might be due not to the disease itself but to the fact that its victims were rendered immobile. He proved the point by recruiting medical students to stay in bed for a month wearing casts that immobilized their lower bodies. Whedon found that the inactivity in these otherwise healthy students caused calcium to leach from their bones. In the early days of the Space Race, Whedon predicted that astronauts would also lose bone calcium because in the near-total absence of gravity in space, they would not need to use their lower limbs. He was right. He also went on to propose bed-rest as the model of choice for studying on the ground the effects of prolonged spaceflight.

The Search for Volunteers

We needed volunteers who were in good health and between twenty-five and fifty-five years old, to match the age of most astronauts. We were honest about the drawbacks. If they joined the experiment they would not be able to have visitors or leave their beds to take a shower or go to the bathroom. And their bodies would undergo changes—which we believed would be reversed once they got up and walked about again. Those who accepted these terms came from many walks of life. Among the volunteers in my studies were some colorful characters: a CIA helicopter pilot, a trombonist, an air-traffic controller, a stand-up comedian, a millionaire, a lawyer, a nurse, an eccentric who had been educated at a private school and was rebelling against society, and a gentle giant of a charmer who kept everyone in order.

Over the years, more than 2,500 men and women have been studied in U.S., Japanese, European, and Russian bed-rest programs. We had surprisingly few dropouts, and only in our earliest studies. The handful that felt they had made the wrong choice came to this decision within three days. We could not, of course, match the excitement of the real thing, but most of our volunteers felt like budding astronauts. They were powerfully motivated by the knowledge that they were making a real contribution to America's space effort. Bed-rest, of course, is no holiday. When I asked volunteers, "What was the hardest part for you?" I expected answers like "the tests," "the diet," or "having to use a bed pan," but the consistent answer was simply "lying in bed."

The Bald facts about Bed-Rest

The success of the U.S. space program in landing men on the Moon led to a reluctant interest by the Soviets in the potential benefits of collaboration. It was a truly historic moment when, in 1975, a U.S. Apollo capsule docked with a Soyuz spacecraft and, for the first time, astronauts and cosmonauts shook hands in space. Soviet and American space scientists got together to share some of their findings and insights. A year later, I visited Moscow with a NASA delegation.

One of our Soviet colleagues, Yuri Sinkevich, told us he had spent thirty days in head-down bed-rest as their first test subject. Sinkovich was an avid collector of new experiences: He was a doctor, a TV personality, a public-relations expert, and, in any time he had left over, an explorer. In 1970, he set out from Africa to cross the Atlantic with the Norwegian explorer Thor Heyerdahl aboard the papyrus raft *Ra II*. Their aim was to demonstrate that ancient people from Africa may have crossed the Atlantic before Columbus. By reaching Barbados in the West Indies they proved their point, in theory at least.

I was interested in getting first-hand impressions about head-down bed-rest from this multi-faceted man. He thought for a bit, then pointed to his bald head, implying that it got that way because of constant rubbing against the headboard. It took me quite a few moments to appreciate his Russian sense of humor.

The Soviets had been in space the longest and they too had decided that the best research method was the one using bed-rest. Towards the early 1970s they improved on this method by tilting the bed so that the head was lower than the feet. This was because returning cosmonauts had complained that lying in a horizontal bed after spaceflight made them feel as though they were slipping off the foot of the bed. The angle of tilt at which they felt most comfortable was six degrees. In 1980, I introduced this Soviet model of head-down bed-rest into the U.S.

Dee O'Hara, already a legend in the U.S. space program, became the manager of NASA's California-based Human Research Facility. As a very young Air Force nurse, she was recruited to be the nurse for the original seven astronauts—Alan Shepard, Scott Carpenter, Gordon Cooper, John Glenn, Gus Grissom, Wally Schirra, and Deke Slayton. She showed amazing skill in handling people of all kinds, from the danger-loving "right stuff" types to the most unassuming of bed-rest volunteers. They respected her and they trusted her, and she stood up for them all. Carrying out these studies for many days was not easy and severely challenged Dee's organizational skills, but she passed with flying colors.

The Case for the Dwarf Payphone

When we wanted a payphone installed in the facility at bedside height, the telephone company told us it was impossible. Payphones could only be fixed at the regulation height—the height suitable for a person who was standing. "But that's not what I want," said Dee O'Hara. "I want it lower."

"Sorry," said the engineer, "I have to follow regulations, so that's what you're going to get." Dee told him this was of no use and indicated with her hand the height at which she wanted the phone. "These guys—they must be dwarfs," said the engineer.

"Oh, but didn't I tell you—that's just what they are," said Dee.

The phone was fixed where she wanted it.

What Did We Learn from This Research?

The bed-rest model proved to be an excellent way of inducing the changes in the body we had seen in astronauts. Granted, they happened more slowly and were less severe than in space. But it was through studying healthy human volunteers lying in bed that we learned how these bodily changes were produced and how they could be prevented.

Just about everybody knows the feelings of dizziness and weakness when getting out of bed after a bout of 'flu. At one time, this was thought to be an aftereffect of the illness. Then similar feelings of wooziness were reported by astronauts from the earliest Mercury and Gemini missions. At first this was believed to be the result of being crammed in the tiny space capsule and seasickness, brought on by bobbing up and down in the ocean after re-entry while waiting to be picked up by helicopter. But we saw similar symptoms—an increased tendency to faint when they finally got out of bed—in our volunteers when they stood up even after as little as twenty-four hours in bed.

Just as in space, blood pressure and the circulation are not alone in being affected by a stay in bed where the effect of gravity is reduced. Muscles, bones, the sense of balance, the digestive system, and the immune system all suffer. One of the most important questions we asked in these studies was how to find ways of preventing these changes in astronauts, especially on long missions.

Is It Just Inactivity That Causes the Problem?

Could exercise, in space or while lying in bed, be the answer? We tested various exercise regimes, including workouts on a kind of horizontal bicycle, and found that they brought about some improvement. But none completely prevented the harmful changes to the human body caused by a reduction in the influence of gravity. The Soviets reported similar disappointing results for a variety of exercise routines, even after turning for advice to the coaches of their Olympic athletes. It was obvious that there was more to these changes than a mere lack of activity. Exercise helps, but it is not the complete solution. Exercise needs gravity to be effective. Using legs to walk requires actively working against the force of gravity.

A Breakthrough in Medical Care

Lying in bed or just sitting around also happen to be what a lot of us do; these are habits that can start as early as the college years. Therefore, anything that helped the astronauts would help anyone leading an increasingly sedentary lifestyle.

The insights from observations in patients, confirmed through our research in healthy people, led to something of a breakthrough in medical and nursing care. Traditionally, patients in hospital were confined to bed for several days even after the mildest surgery in the belief that rest would help recovery. After a hernia operation, childbirth, or a routine appendectomy, patients would commonly spend seven to ten days in bed. Now hernias are done as an outpatient procedure and the others normally involve one- or two-day stays.

Getting people up and about as soon as possible after surgery is now considered good practice. It has been adopted because it accelerates recovery and healing. This is one of the best examples of how not using gravity properly (lying in bed) can delay recovery. On the other hand, using it effectively (standing and walking, even with help) is beneficial. Health-insurance companies were quick to endorse these findings.

Staying Young and Healthy

If astronauts do not grow old faster in space, why do they return to Earth showing so many of the symptoms we associate with aging? The similarities between the changes produced in astronauts in space and in men and women lying in bed right here on Earth led to many intriguing questions. Were our volunteers growing "old" simply by lying in bed? Clearly not. Both our volunteers and astronauts recovered fully after getting up and about on Earth's gravity. What was going on? The simplistic answer was that the symptoms may seem similar but are in fact due to different mechanisms. After all, as the received wisdom goes, we all know that they are not reversible in the elderly—or so we have been led to believe.

What "Aging" Can Mean—and What It *Should* Mean

In the midst of one of my bed-rest studies in California, I had an opportunity to observe some of the problems of aging firsthand. The mother of some good friends of mine fell and broke her hip. She was in her late seventies and needed full-time care, which could only be provided in a nursing home in nearby San Jose. For me it was a whole new world.

When I visited the home, I found that some of the residents lay in bed or sat in the lobby at what seemed like the same spot, day in day out, staring blankly ahead. A few occasionally struggled down the hall with a walker. Most ate or drank very little and even had trouble raising a fork to their mouths and chewing. Few were reading. All looked very frail and showed no interest in their surroundings. While talking to the staff I was told some were rarely, if ever, visited. Their muscles got weaker. If they fell over, because their sense of balance was so poor, their broken bones did not seem to heal. In fact, most never recovered after a hip fracture. These changes were assumed to be the permanent and irreversible results of age. It was disheartening—a one-way street, despite all the valiant efforts of the staff. This, I thought, is what aging means for far too many people.

The All-Important Question: Can "Aging" Be Reversed?

I had done many bed-rest studies before and was well aware of the changes produced. But it was not until I visited the nursing home that it dawned on me that the question should perhaps be turned around. It was not "Do astronauts and bed-rest volunteers grow old under conditions of reduced gravity?" What if the question I had to ask was "Could the physical deterioration so obvious in the people in the nursing home be caused by some factor other than the unavoidable accumulation of years? Could it have something to do with gravity?" The answer to this question raised a highly exciting prospect.

Redefining the Concept of Aging

The more I looked into the matter, the more convinced I became that many of the symptoms of aging had little to do with which birthday you last celebrated. The theory I developed was that they are due to the gradual reduction, over many, many years—perhaps a lifetime—of the influence of gravity on the human body. "But," you may say, "gravity is all around us. We live in it our entire lives. How can it be good for some things and bad for others? If it is supposed to be a force for good, how can it make me stoop and look older?"

Clearly, the force of gravity does not change. It must, therefore, be something we do, or stop doing, that makes the difference to our bodies. And for most of us, the main lifestyle change as the years go by is that we start to take things easy. We are encouraged by friends, family, and others around us to rest, or even retire. The result is that we make less and less use of gravity. Yes, gravity is always present, but if we do not use it, what good is it? People who adopt an easier life-style are, in effect, taking shelter from gravity. Like the astronauts and my volunteers, they develop the symptoms we have come to associate with old age, as the dictionary defines it.

On Earth, we are constantly exposed to some gravity, however little we use it, so the changes take a lifetime to become evident or serious. People who avoid using gravity will age much faster than those who develop good gravity-challenging habits early on and keep them up throughout the rest of their lives. Understanding gravity and developing good gravity-challenging habits is the secret for aging well.

Challenging Gravity/Understanding a Difficult Concept

Gravity does not just make apples fall off trees. It keeps us firmly grounded and gives "weight" to our body mass. Body weight is a very important factor in our lives. It provides the load that stimulates structures that support us, such as bones and muscles. When you are standing up or sitting, your arms naturally hang down by your sides. That is because gravity is pulling them down. If you raise an arm in front of you, you must exert some effort to keep it there. You are challenging gravity.

You will soon find that your arm feels heavy and tired. If for some reason your muscles have become weak, as happens after a bone fracture or illness, you may have trouble keeping your arm up for very long. If you are also holding something, such as a tea cup or a jug of water, you may find it difficult to keep it steady. Exercises with handheld weights use gravity to strengthen muscles. Japanese astronaut Chiaki Mukai tells of her amazement after returning from her first mission, when she put a piece of paper on her outstretched hand. "It was SO...OOH heavy!" she says.

In space with almost no gravity, the arms of astronauts do not hang by their sides but seem to float in front of them. They do not stand on the floor because there is no up or down. Their feet are off the floor, legs slightly bent because they have no weight to carry. Their head leans forward because it does not need to be supported by the spine for balance. Astronauts do not need to put on their pants one leg at a time, but they soon learn it is faster to put both legs in at the same time.

We challenge gravity all the time in little ways—combing our hair, pointing at something, chewing, getting in and out of a car, carrying bags of groceries, holding a baby. We challenge gravity in more rigorous ways when we get out of bed, climb a ladder, walk up a hill, go up or down stairs, or jump. Even standing challenges gravity, because we are resisting its pull, moving in the opposite direction to its force. "But," you may say, "standing is not moving." If you think of moving as something beyond changing location—something that requires you to make an effort, to contract some muscle—then merely standing fits that bill. Think of it this way. If when you stood up you went absolutely limp and did not contract any muscles at all, you would crumble to the floor in a heap. Gravity would pull you there. Not only do you need to contract muscles to move your body up, but you continue to contract muscles to remain standing, even though most of us are not aware of the effort.

Rudolf Nureyev and Mikhail Baryshnikov, the Russian ballet dancers, were spectacular when they jumped because they seemed stationary, suspended in mid-air. Michael Jordan often appeared to do the same thing. It was their energy and powerful muscles that kept them there longer than the average person, despite gravity pulling them down. In fact, they were defying gravity. High jumpers break records in much the same way. Ordinary jumping, or just standing, similarly challenges gravity. Lifting a hand weight by curling your arm challenges gravity and tones up the muscle that does the curling—the biceps. But think of the way down—most people simply drop their arm, giving in to gravity and receiving no benefit. However, if you make the same motion *very slowly*, resisting gravity, the benefits of this exercise are far greater, for you will be toning up your triceps, as well. Becoming aware of how you use gravity in everything you do allows you to use it to your advantage.

We are not all Nureyevs—nor do we need to be. Every little thing we do can either take advantage of gravity or be a waste of a good opportunity. Consider the benefits of sitting upright in a chair against slumping in a sofa. Or of walking up and down the stairs instead of using the elevator. These examples demonstrate how in simple everyday activities we can either take advantage of gravity or be a gravity dodger.

Start Investing in Yourself

You may say, "I don't regard myself as old, I'm no couch potato, I exercise regularly, and I certainly don't spend too much time in bed. So why should I worry?" This may well be so, but have you ever totted up exactly how much of the day you spend at an office desk or sitting in front of a computer, and how much of the evening you lounge in front of the TV screen? Or have you considered how much time you spend in your car instead of walking? Even if you go to the gym for an hour each day, it is not enough, unless you are consciously using gravity to stimulate every part of your body the rest of the time.

All exercise, all movement, is good for the body. Deliberate movements that use gravity as a comprehensive stimulus bring the maximum benefits. And if you develop a set of habits in your life based on this approach, you are well on your way to building up a fund of health and vigor. In effect, you will be making a valuable long-term investment in yourself.

Why is it important to invest in yourself? Think of it as building up a nest egg for the future, in exactly the same way that you set aside regular savings to draw on when you retire. When you are no longer generating the same income as when you were working, this nest egg will help you maintain your standard of living at the very period when you have more time to enjoy life.

Even if you saved, the value of your savings will decline over time if you do not invest them. This is what happens to our vitality—call it youth, if you will—as well. How can you prevent this decline? By investing in yourself. This depends on embarking on a regular health savings-and-investment program by consciously developing habits that use gravity effectively. You can build up your reserves of health and vigor so that they will be there whenever you need them, for as long as you live. You can maintain your bone and muscle strength, good balance and coordination, youthful spring, enthusiasm, curiosity, and that twin-kle in your eye that says you are always ready for new adventures.

Will this approach extend your life? Perhaps. Will it prevent disease? Possibly. There is no evidence either way other than the evidence provided by your own eyes, but it stands to reason that if you keep yourself healthy with a diverse grav-ity-harnessing portfolio, you will be less likely to suffer from a great number of diseases discussed in this book. Investing in yourself will certainly give you what you need to carry on doing the things you enjoy.

Gravity Is a Total Package

Harnessing the power of gravity is a way of life. Understanding how we use grav-ity to keep ourselves in tip-top shape, both physically and emotionally, is the first step. Keep using it and your body will readjust to a new and higher level of func-tion. Your sensors will regain their sharpness to respond. Your support structures will be strengthened by the load of the body's mass—the body's weight. Your hormone and immune systems will react positively to stress. You will sleep better. You will feel good and full of energy. You will enjoy what you eat, see, smell, and taste to a greater degree. Every system in the body, and its ability to respond to external challenges, depends on the way we use the gravity that surrounds us. Gravity is a total and comprehensive package.

We do not have all the answers. I chose the systems in the chapters that follow as examples because we have direct and obvious evidence of how gravity affects them. But the body consists of many interdependent systems. Like a good orches-tra, it makes beautiful music when its parts work in harmony.

Professional musicians are naturally talented, but it is only through hard and constant practice that they achieve peak performance. However accomplished they may be individually, it takes rehearsal and the conductor to achieve a perfect symphony. So it is with our bodies. Gravity is the stimulus for each system and the catalyst for the whole—it is the key ingredient.

What Follows

The following chapters outline what we now know about the way the body works. They provide information to help you understand how we constantly use gravity as a stimulus. You will come to know what happens in space, when gravity is minimized, and on Earth, when we do not use it fully due to bad habits that we develop over the years. At the end of each chapter is a section covering the merits or drawbacks of remedies for the conditions that result from our misuse of gravity. This will provide the information you need to make smart choices. Most of these remedies are currently available. Others are still in the research stage.

Breaking the Myth

Every sense and every system in your body—every bone, muscle, tissue, fiber, and cell—withers or thrives according to the way in which you use gravity. This book challenges the widely-held belief that many of the changes associated with aging are unavoidable. We cannot stop the passing of years, but we can certainly halt and even reverse what comes with it. No one is beyond repair.

Some people trying to lose weight put a picture of an obese person on the refrigerator door to discourage themselves from raiding its contents. However young and healthy you may now be, think ahead to how you might look and feel a few years or decades down the road if you neglect to make full use of gravity. Hermann Doernemann, Germany's oldest man, put it well when he said on his 110th birthday, "If I had known I was going to live this long, I would have taken better care of myself."

The Support Structures

Bones, muscles, joints, and skin encase the body, hold it together, support it, and enable us to move around. They are all collagen based. A fibrous protein, collagen is what gives elasticity and resilience to these tissues. Collagen fibers are flexible because they are joined together by small crosslinks that allow the fibers to slide up and down. If these crosslinks are damaged by injury or stiffened by inflammation, poor diet, or age, the flexibility of the collagen fibers will be limited, causing, among other things, feelings of stiffness in the joints and thinner, less elastic skin. Problems also arise when collagen is broken down by the enzyme collagenase and is not renewed.

We do not know exactly how support structures sense gravity, but they do respond to "loading." The load in this case is our body's weight. Bones in obese people are thicker and stronger. Without the loading provided by gravity, bones, muscles, and collagen will atrophy in organs that support the body's weight.

In the near-zero gravity of space the body has no weight, so bones, muscles, and joints do not have to carry a load. They are, therefore, deprived of the stimulus required to grow and thrive in order to hold up the body. As there is no signal, the body concludes that no response is needed. Something similar happens over a longer time to people down here on Earth, who use gravity less and less by leading inactive lives or who cannot sense its force because of injury to the spine or brain.

Although a great deal of research on how unloading in space affects muscles and bones has been carried out, no studies have been done on the skin and very few on the joints of astronauts.

2

Load Your Bones

o o o o o o o o o o o o o o o o o o o o o o o o o o o o o o o o o o

Full fathom five thy father lies;
Of his bones are coral made;
Those are pearls that were his eyes;
Nothing of him that doth fade,
But doth suffer a sea-change
Into something rich and strange.

—William Shakespeare (1564–1616), The Tempest

There are more than 200 bones in the human body, providing both the internal scaffolding that supports it and the levers that help it move. Durable as they are, compared with other parts of the body, bones deteriorate and change as we grow older—not into something particularly rich and strange but into something frailer and more brittle than they were in youth.

Teenagers and twenty-something-year-olds can emerge from the rough and tumble of contact sports, or from a fall, with just a bruise or two. If they break a bone it heals within two weeks. But if an elderly person falls over, the chances of a bone fracture are fairly high. Nearly 90% of all fractures in the elderly are caused by falls. A large number die within a year of the fracture. This is not due to the fracture but to being bedridden. However, there are ways of slowing down the rate at which bones deteriorate and of delaying the onset of the process. All of them involve the harnessing of gravity as an ally. This is the lesson we have learned from space.

Waiting for the Boys to Get Back

Pauline Beery Mack, a professor at Texas Women's University, in Denton, was passionately concerned about the dangers of weakening bones in early astronauts. There were then no fancy laboratories at NASA's landing sites to measure the changes in Gemini and Apollo astronauts. She was known to sit on an orange crate "waiting for [her] boys" to return from their missions, so she could measure the changes in their bone density. At the time there were no sensitive bone-densitometry methods either. X-rays were the best we had. Detecting bone loss was very much an art.

Yet she was convinced she detected losses in density of 1–3% in the heel bone. Why the heel bone? Because the heel carries the bulk of the body's load on Earth; thus, it was expected to be the first to show changes when it no longer had to carry that load in space.

Why You Wake Up Taller

When our remote ancestors first began to stand upright, they were taking on an extra burden of gravity. Bones, muscles, joints, and the ligaments and tendons that interconnect them had to evolve in new ways in order to support the upright body and to enable human beings to move freely and work in gravity. Its compressive force on the spinal column, pelvis, leg joints, and heels is so powerful that we go to bed at night one-half to one centimeter shorter than when we get up in the morning. When the stimulus of gravity is, in effect, removed altogether, the body length of an astronaut can increase by two to five centimeters during a spaceflight of just five days.

In addition to the direct compressive influence of gravity on the spine and leg bones, the pull of muscles on the various bone structures to which they are attached provides indirect loading on the skeleton. If unchallenged, this compressive force of gravity will result in our getting shorter as we age. In contrast, harnessing gravity to stimulate support structures can prevent this compression and all its associated problems, such as painful slipped discs.

Bones in the Language

Bones have given a wealth of expressions to the language. Somebody who is incorrigibly lazy is "bone-idle." Insult somebody's intelligence and you might describe him or her as "a bonehead." If you fall out with somebody, you have "a bone to pick" with your opponent. An issue that leads to disputes between nations or between other groups can become "a bone of contention." Those who wish to speak frankly, or even rudely, on a topic will "make no bones about it." An ambitious mobster, on the other hand, will "make his bones" by eliminating somebody who has betrayed or in some other way angered his boss. If you want to master a subject quickly, just before an examination for instance, you will "bone up on it." An embarrassing mistake is a "boner." It is said of hard drinkers, heavy smokers, or people who hit the night spots too often that they will "never make old bones." If you have a premonition that something is about to happen, or a sensation not supported by direct evidence, you "feel it in your bones."

How the System Works

Much as studying tree rings can tell us a great deal about the life of the tree, so can the appearance of bone tissue speak volumes about the life of a human being. If you cut across a leg bone, you can see rings where new bone has been deposited during years of growth. The central hollow houses bone marrow. For many years, it was believed that bone is a relatively inert structure. After all, it is the only part of the body that, for centuries, can survive the decay of death. In fact, we can lose bone quite rapidly while we are alive. It is only in the last sixty years that bone has been recognized as a highly dynamic tissue. In addition to forming the structural support for the body, bone is a major player in maintaining the right balance of calcium and other minerals.

A New You—Every Ten Years

For most of our lives, our skeletons go through a continuous process of destruction and rebuilding. This is so extensive that scientists have calculated that the adult skeleton is completely regenerated every ten years. Bone mass is critical for bone strength and durability. If the bone mass is low, the bones will become brittle and easily broken. More than 90% of the body's calcium is contained in bones, and only 0.08 % in the bloodstream; the rest is found in organs, such as the kidneys and intestines.

A constant exchange of calcium between bones and the blood is of critical importance to life. This exchange is regulated by hormones and by vitamin D. Too little calcium in the blood and muscles will not pick up signals to contract—so the heart, for instance, could stop beating. Too much can result in kidney stones, depression, uraemic poisoning, and, at worst, death. If the regulation of blood calcium goes even mildly wrong, the symptoms, though less severe, will still be unpleasant.

The balance is upset in cases of parathyroidism, the production by the parathyroid gland of a hormone that causes calcium levels in the blood to increase. The consequences, as spelled out by the American Society for Bone and Mineral Research, are "easy fatigability, a sense of weakness, and a feeling that the aging process is advancing faster than it should." Parathyroidism is sometimes accompanied by "an intellectual weariness and a sense that cognitive faculties are less sharp." These symptoms may sound familiar to many of us, but who would have suspected that bones and calcium levels could have possibly been one of the reasons?

The Structure of Bones

Bones are characterized by an impressive combination of strength and lightness. The longer tubular bones of the limbs are stronger than steel yet only one third its weight. The material from which bone is made is collagen, the fibrous protein in which are embedded microscopic particles of calcium, phosphorous, and other minerals, including trace elements of copper and cobalt. Collagen is also the home of cells that make and break down bone.

There are two different kinds of bone tissue: compact, or *cortical bone*, which is tough and dense; and cancellous, or *trabecular bone*, which has a spongy texture and a honeycomb-like structure. Trabecular bone, so named from the Latin *trabecula*, meaning small beam, consists of thin rods of bony tissue embedded in spongy bone. These rods form a mesh of interconnected spaces that contain the bone marrow. Trabecular bone is found mainly in the spine and makes up about 15% of the bone in the body. The dense and compact cortical bone, making up the remaining 85%, is found in such parts of the skeleton as the skull, the hips, the long bones of the arms and legs, and the outer shell of flat bones, such as the shoulder blades.

How Bone Is Created—and Destroyed

Both types of bone tissue contain three types of cells: osteoblasts, osteocytes, and osteoclasts. The *osteoblasts* (from two Greek words meaning "bone" and "shoot" or "bud") constantly form new bone by manufacturing a protein matrix, a three-dimensional network of cells that becomes calcified as it lays down new bone material. *Osteoclasts* (from "bone" and "breakage") balance this process by breaking down bone in a process called resorption. *Osteocytes* ("bone" and "hollow vessel"), the most common cells in bone, are osteoblasts encased in mineral and are believed to be the cells that sense loading, the pull of gravity and of the muscles on bone. When a bone is fractured, blood clots form between the broken fragments. Osteoblast cells move to the site of damage to form new tissue. Osteoclast cells dissolve and sculpt the new tissue as necessary so that the bone recovers its original shape.

In healthy people, there is a constant balance between the two processes of creating and destroying bone tissue, but if this balance is upset, the results can be calamitous. At one extreme comes the severe bone loss of *osteoporosis*, where resorption exceeds formation and bones become more brittle. At the other extreme lies the rare disease of *osteopetrosis* (meaning "rock hard"), in which the bones become too dense and lose their bending properties.

The constant remodeling of bone to maintain its integrity, strength, and density depends heavily on loading—the mechanical forces applied to the skeleton when it supports the body's weight and responds to the stresses and strains created by movement. Muscles pull on the bones at attachment sites, stimulating an increase in density near those sites. In this way, internal loading determines the architecture of bone so that it is more dense in some parts than in others.

The Role of Hormones, Steroids, and Vitamins

A number of hormones play key roles in either bone formation or bone loss. On the positive side, the sex hormones, estrogen in women and testosterone in men, are essential for the proper development and maintenance of healthy bone. Growth hormone is needed for proper bone development in children and for the maximum positive effect of loading on bone in adults.

On the negative side, increased levels of steroids (corticosteroids, such as cortisol) can aggravate bone loss. These hormones are secreted by the adrenal gland in response to stress or depression, or they are prescribed as a treatment for arthritis or allergies. Diseases of the thyroid, or of the parathyroid gland that lead to the production of large amounts of parathyroid hormone (PTH), can also lead to bone loss. PTH and vitamin D affect bone by regulating calcium. A modest decrease in the level of calcium in the blood when calcium intake is inadequate is rapidly followed by an increase in PTH. This forces bone to give up calcium and kidneys to conserve calcium, so that its level in the blood is restored within a few hours. Vitamin D is needed for the intestines to absorb calcium. Herrings, salmon, tuna, liver, and egg yolk are all good sources of this vitamin, and exposure to daylight is crucial to its synthesis in the skin.

As we grow older, the cycle of building and shedding bone tends to shift out of balance. Bone mass can be lost faster than it is built for many natural reasons: changes in hormone levels, insufficient calcium intake in the diet or a reduction in its absorption, reduced time spent outdoors, or a less active lifestyle. Space-flight has a similar effect, but at a faster rate. Research using unloading in space and bed-rest here on Earth has been useful in suggesting and testing remedies for the deterioration in bone we associate with aging.

Overweight People Have Stronger Bones, but...

The state of adult bone, its density and strength, are determined by its loading history. The load on the body or body-weight depends on gravity, without which we would have mass but no weight. An astronaut on the Moon weighs only one sixth of what he weighs on Earth, because of the lower gravity there. On Earth, doubling one's mass also doubles the weight and the load on the skeleton. Because of this increased loading, obese individuals have a higher bone density than smaller or thinner people. They are therefore less likely to break a bone when they fall.

The bad news is that the increased weight compresses the joints of knees and hips, and correcting these problems often requires surgery. Being overweight results in other serious health drawbacks too, such as the risk of high blood pressure, heart attacks, and diabetes.

It is not necessary to be overweight to increase loading on bones. You can increase the load on your leg bones by wearing weights around your ankles when you exercise or walk. If you are already a senior, you can at the very least hang on to what you have. You can reduce your rate of bone loss through outdoor activities such as walking, tennis, or dancing. Remaining physically active is a healthier way to achieve the same result. For example, the weight borne by your heels when you are standing (1G) can be increased by 20% when you walk (1.2G). It increases threefold (3G) when you jog and up to six-fold (6G) if you jump.

During the years of childhood and puberty, loading effects are amplified by the surge of developmental hormones, growth hormone, and sex hormones that build up muscle and bone. New bone is formed faster than old bone is broken down. Along with the size of muscles, the density and strength of bone continues to increase, peaking at around twenty to thirty years of age. After that age, the average rate of bone loss is calculated to be around 1% a year. But people have been known to live to around 120, by which age they would have no bones at all if that rate of loss applied; and a man of eighty would have only half the bone mass he had at thirty. This average figure of 1% bone loss a year means there are many who are losing bone at a much faster rate. It also includes some very active people, who lose bone at a much slower rate and tend to live healthier, longer lives.

There is no question that an active life delays and diminishes bone loss. But an increasing number of people are not too diligent about remaining active. Dr. Alexandre Kalache, coordinator of the Aging and Health Program of the World Health Organization, calculates that the denser your bones are at the peak of growth (around the mid-twenties), the longer you are likely to enjoy strong bones. It pays, then, to take up active sports when you are young and to keep them up as you grow older. You can certainly play a role in influencing youngsters in your family to get out and about and build up their bone reserves while they can. It is the best investment in their future health and independence.

What Can Go Wrong?

Unloading Bone

When an astronaut goes into space, or when somebody on Earth sits down, lies down, or spends a lot of time in water, bone is unloaded. The expression "taking a load off your feet" best describes what is meant by unloading. An extreme example of adaptation to unloading is seen in the animal kingdom, in the evolution of sea mammals such as whales and dolphins. The bulk of their weight is supported by the sea so that they are essentially "weightless." Over the eons their skeletons evolved to the point where they have only vestiges of legs. If humans spend much of their lives off their feet, bones no longer need to support the body's full weight, so they respond to signals that they are no longer needed and reduce their strength and density. The body lays down less new bone and starts losing old bone at a rate in keeping with its new loading level.

Your Bones Have a Memory

Although unloading eventually causes bone loss throughout the skeleton, its effects are most evident in bones that normally play the greatest role in supporting the body's weight. Studies of patients who are up and about, but have one leg immobilized so that it does not bear weight, show bone loss only in that leg. Sara Arnaud at NASA's Ames Research Center in California reports that "during spaceflight, bone loss is highly localized. Weight-bearing bones are affected, but no losses have been found in bones in the upper extremities. Bone responds to reduced mechanical loads in space and on Earth during bed-rest." She goes on to list the factors that determine how bone will respond when gravity is removed. They include the previous load and activity of the bone, the age and nutrition of the astronaut, and the output of hormones. In this way bone can be thought to "store" the memory of what it was like to be loaded. This memory makes recovery possible, once the bone has been reloaded. The longer bone remains unloaded, the more likely it is that this memory will be lost, and the less likely it is to recover.

Pedaling in Space Gets the Astronauts Nowhere

Unloading also affects bones indirectly by weakening the muscles attached to them. Muscle loss in space precedes measurable bone loss by about eleven days. The bone loss decreases first at sites of attachment of the muscles that atrophy most. Uneven loss of bone cells changes the architecture of the bone while in space.

The traditional exercises performed by astronauts in space, such as pedaling on a bicycle ergometer, have not prevented bone loss, even if carried out for two to four hours a day. Walking on a treadmill in space while held down with bungee cords produces only a fraction of the loading on the bones one would find on Earth. Calculations by Peter Cavanagh and his group at the Cleveland Clinic estimate that such loading is at best not even equivalent to half their body-weight. It is likely, however, that the bone loss might have been still greater had the astronauts not exercised at all.

Shannon Lucid, who spent six months on the Russian space station *Mir* in 1996, exercised methodically on the treadmill even though running was never her favorite activity on Earth. Though the exact amount of bone she lost is protected by the Privacy Act, it took over two years for her bone to return to the slower rate of loss she had on Earth before this long flight.

Calcium Loss

Whether bone is unloaded as a result of space travel, lying in bed, or just too much sitting around, the loss shows up as a negative calcium balance. This means more calcium is excreted in the urine, feces, and sweat than is taken in through the diet. The major source of such calcium loss is the bone. In space, calcium in the urine increases from the first day of unloading, and the negative calcium balance reaches a peak at about five weeks. A net loss in bone mineral can be measured in weight-bearing bones, primarily the legs and spine.

Over several months of unloading, resorption (the process of breaking down bone tissue) returns to normal, but bone formation remains suppressed. For those people who experience the longest periods of unloading, calcium balance is restored to normal after six to eighteen months, but by that time they will have already lost a significant amount of bone and be very fragile.

The same thing happens to paraplegics, paralyzed by spinal cord damage. Lost ground is not made up as long as the bones sense no load. Paraplegics often break bones because they cannot feel where their limbs are. An arm or leg can get twisted and broken before they realize what has happened. Many people have at one time or another had the experience of an arm or leg "going to sleep" and have fallen or twisted a limb when they tried to use it.

A Week in Space Can Cause as Much Bone Loss as a Year on Earth

In bed-rest, the calcium loss peaks at about 150 mg a day. This corresponds to losing 0.5% of total body calcium every day, resulting in a loss of bone mass. Similarly, in patients paralyzed by spinal-cord injury there is a negative calcium balance corresponding to a daily loss of approximately 0.33% of total body calcium. In space, calcium loss is far greater. It peaks at around 0.8% of total body calcium a day and the calcium balance is still negative after eighty-four days of flight. The average bone loss in Soviet cosmonauts, recorded on missions of four to ten months on Space Station *Mir*, was of the order of 2% to 3% a week, though it has been as low as 0.5% a week in some individuals. This bone loss was discovered by scanning their thigh bones (femurs) and hip joints before and after the flight.

What these findings tell us is that in space, where there is practically no loading of hips and leg bones, the amount of bone lost every week is just shy of what is lost every year here on Earth as we age.

Are Astronauts at Risk of Bone Fractures

It stands to reason that astronauts, some of whom have lost as much as 30% of their bone density in space, must be at a much higher risk of breaking a bone. However, NASA's Linda Shackelford at the Johnson Space Center, in Texas, admits that if compared to other men and women in their age group, the bone density of returning astronauts is about 97% of that normal range. How could that be? It turns out that they are so fit before going into space that their bone density could be as high as 130% greater than their contemporaries from the general population. These much higher bone-density levels in the astronaut population emphasize the value of exercise in increasing bone density above normal levels.

A New Scanner That Leads to More Accurate Measurement

One of the handicaps in understanding bone dynamics has been that scanning methods have not been sufficiently sensitive to catch the changes early. Nor have the scanning techniques told us about changes in bone architecture. Thomas Lang at the University of California, San Francisco, is using a new kind of scanning device—quantitative computed tomography (QCT)—that provides detailed information about the distribution of bone loss. He used it on the crew of seven men and one woman (five of them American and three Russian), who spent periods of four to five and a half months on the International Space Station from 2000 to 2003. Lang recorded a bone loss of 8% in the femur. This is about the same as the measurement taken previously on the Soviet spaceship *Mir*. However, with the sensitive QCT, the sites of greatest change could be identified. He found that the honeycombed trabecular bone in the head of the femur—the part that fits into the hip socket and is closest to muscle-attachment sites—lost as much as 12% of its bone-mineral density. On the other hand, the loss of hard cortical bone in the interior of the bone was only 4%. This disproportionate loss makes the femur head more vulnerable to fracture.

Unloading also weakens the adhesion of tendons and ligaments to bone by causing a breakdown of collagen. The cushioning ability of discs between the vertebrae of the spine is reduced, and connective tissue may move in to fill the spaces between them. Protruding slipped discs and back pain are common in astronauts after spaceflight, when the weight of the body makes the vertebrae collapse on each other because of weakened back muscles that support the spine and inadequate cushioning between them. They recover by doing exercises to strengthen their back muscles and relieve the pressure of the body's weight on the vertebrae.

Great care is taken during the rehabilitation of astronauts, who are anxious to return to the high level of fitness they enjoyed before going into space. They weight train in small, steady increments and when they begin supervised walking back on Earth, they start slowly and increase speed gradually to avoid tearing muscles and ligaments.

Anyone who has spent a long period in bed—because of illness, injury, or surgery, for example—needs similar care. Such care after a period of unloading is especially important for older patients.

Wear + Tear + Neglect = Arthritis

But you do not have to be old or spend a long time in bed to feel aches and pains. Who has not experienced tenderness in the soles of their feet or in their ankles and hips when they first get out of bed in the morning? Dare I say this can happen as early as in your fifties? It can come from idleness or abuse, such as jogging on a hard surface.

Aches, pain, swelling, and stiffness in the joints, muscles, bones, and connective tissues, such as tendons and ligaments, are generally symptoms of arthritis, or they are the early signs of the wear and tear that leads to arthritis. It can strike at any age, child or adult. The most common type, osteoarthritis, affects more than 21 million Americans. It causes the degeneration of cartilage so they suffer the agony of bone grinding against bone. Another two million suffer from rheumatoid arthritis, in which the body's own immune system attacks joints, often damaging both bone and cartilage and causing pain and inflammation. Bursitis (also known as tennis elbow or housemaid's knee, depending on its site) and tendonitis have symptoms similar to those of arthritis but result from injury or overuse and are more easily treatable.

Effects of the Menopause

Dramatic changes in hormone output of the kind experienced by women during the menopause may further accelerate the rate of bone loss. The rate of loss is similar in both men and women except during the few years around menopause, when the normal output of female hormones decreases. The average age of menopause in the U.S. is 51.4 years, but it can happen any time between 40 and 60. Some women may lose no bone at all. Most lose up to 5% of bone mass per year for the three to five years that the change of life lasts. After that, the loss returns to its pre-menopause rate. Women who go through a more gradual menopause later in life are likely to be affected less than those for whom the change is more sudden. After the menopause, and as a result of weakened abdominal, back, and neck muscles, and poor posture, some women can develop a curvature of the spine that is known as a "dowager's hump." This is because the spongy trabecular bone, which forms the spine, loses its cells faster than hard cortical bone is lost in other parts of the skeleton.

Women on hormone replacement therapy (HRT) who stop their medication abruptly are also more likely to lose bone at a faster rate than those who gradually taper off their HRT. As estrogen levels diminish with the beginning of menopause, estrogen replacement, using slow-release skin patches, can reduce the bone loss. One of the stages that can precede osteoporosis is a condition known as osteopenia—low bone density. Women identified as having smaller bones when they are aged twenty-five to thirty usually get this condition earlier than those with larger bones. Men have fewer problems with bone loss, because their bones are bigger to begin with than those of women and because they go through a more gradual decrease in their hormone output, which comes at a later age.

Hip Fractures: Women Are at Greater Risk

Women who have passed the menopause have a three-fold greater risk of fracture than men of the same age because their rate of bone loss is greater. The pattern of loss is very different between the sexes, with women experiencing greater loss of bone strength in the spine and hips. The National Institute on Aging reports that by about age 50, 17.5% of women and 6% of men will have had a hip fracture and 15.6% of women as compared with 5% of men will have suffered fractures of the vertebrae. By age 80, half of all women will have broken the head of a femur or a vertebra. For every man who suffers a vertebral fracture, six women have the same harrowing experience. In the U.S. alone, there are 350,000 hip fractures every year requiring hospitalization and extensive rehabilitation, while incurring great cost and pain.

The Scourge of Osteoporosis

Imagine bones so weak, so brittle, so leached of calcium and riddled with holes that they begin to look like Gruyère cheese. You are looking at the final stage of the disease of osteoporosis. It afflicts many people, not just the elderly, and causes a change in bone architecture and a greater reduction in bone mass than osteopenia, the bone loss that most people experience with passing years. Unloading of the bones clearly makes osteoporosis worse. But this condition is sometimes found in very active people, indicating there is more to the disease than just inactivity.

Ten million people in the United States that we know of currently suffer from osteoporosis and the World Health Organization estimates that there are 250 million cases in the world. There is a 50-50 chance of becoming a victim once you have passed the age of 75. It is even greater in some women after menopause so that three out of every four osteoporosis sufferers are women.

Osteoporosis increases the risk of a fracture—a risk that doubles for every 10% of bone loss. In the U.S. it is believed to be responsible each year for 1.3 million bone fractures in the elderly. Most are in the spine (700,000), hip (300,000) or wrist (250,000). They occur predominantly among Caucasians and Asians, for African Americans tend to have stronger bones. As the U.S. population ages over the next 20 years, the incidence of fractures is expected to double if no effective treatment for osteoporosis is found. It is equally important to develop much more sensitive and inexpensive methods of earlier detection and of tracking changes in the bones before fractures happen.

The Centers for Disease Control in Atlanta warn that hip fractures in the elderly increase the risk of dying by 24% in just the first year. It is not so much the shock of the fracture that brings about a rapid decline in health as the immobilization that follows. It also has an emotional impact because people lose their independence.

Feelings of stress and depression sometimes lead to osteoporosis, because they send the adrenal glands, located above the kidneys, into overdrive, and the extra steroids churning through the bloodstream can accelerate the loss of bone tissue and suppress the formation of new bone.

Other Risk Factors

Other diseases that affect bone and become more common as we age are related to inflammation. Rheumatoid arthritis, sometimes called osteoarthritis, is such a disease. It is painful because it destroys the collagen in cartilage, the 'padding' in the joints, so that bone grinds directly on bone, causing excessive erosion.

Many factors can promote bone loss–among them genetic predisposition or early menopause. Heavy smoking, drinking more than two cups of coffee, or more than two glasses of wine a day, may also make you lose bone faster. Smoking is toxic to osteoblasts (the cells that build bone), and if you look at heavy smokers, especially women, they are usually thin and have early menopause. Smoking may also reduce the beneficial effects of HRT. Excessive salt in the diet– or too little chromium, copper or magnesium—can also accelerate bone loss.

The Acid Theory

New research suggests that excess acid in the body may be linked to the rise in osteoporosis in the west. Tim Arnett at University College, London, proposed that our cells work best if they are not exposed to an acidic environment. Even a slight shift to a more acid pH in the blood tells the body to draw on more alkaline calcium from the bones to neutralize it. People taking bicarbonate of soda for excessive acid stomachs were found to have stronger bones. Arnett believes that future research may substantiate his thesis that some antacids may protect bones from excessive calcium loss. Research at the Swiss drug company Novartis, have identified acid receptors in bone cells. Acid levels may be the primary signal to make osteoclasts more active in breaking down bone.

What makes blood more acid? A diet rich in animal fats, cheese and wheat will raise blood acid levels. In contrast, fruit and vegetables make blood more alkaline after they are metabolized. Chewing the antacid tablets TUMS (calcium carbonate) was popular as a source of calcium some years ago and may have done double duty by making blood more alkaline as well. As we age kidneys become less efficient at excreting acid in the urine. Poor blood flow to bone caused by inflammation, diseased blood vessels or a sedentary lifestyle also cause a shift to greater acidity that probably contribute to bone loss in all these conditions.

High levels of carbon dioxide in an enclosed space also raise blood acidity and can promote bone loss. Sitting in a room with an open fire that burns the oxygen can increase the carbon dioxide in the room if there is inadequate ventilation. So too, in a spaceship, where there is no convection, exhaled carbon dioxide may build up if ventilation is poor. On Earth, soda-pop especially those with caffeine and colas that are very acid also contribute to bone loss.

Though protein in the diet is a good way of building strong bones, too much of it can have the opposite effect. Weight loss diets that depend on a high protein intake can lead to bone loss. Many weight loss diets are not balanced and cause a form of malnutrition. Malnutrition in general and too much weight loss will also increase bone loss. Norm Thagard, the first U.S. astronaut on the Russian station *Mir*, lost 37.4 lbs (17Kg) of his body weight and more bone during his flight than his fellow crew-members because he did not eat enough. Once in the near-zero gravity of space, his appetite diminished—especially for the Soviet space diet, rich in canned fish which are good sources of calcium.

Rebuilding Bone

It is very difficult to rebuild bone. After spaceflight or bed-rest, even though healthy adults begin to rebuild bone as soon as their bodies are fully loaded again by gravity, recovery is very slow. From observations based on limited data, it appears that bone loss in space stops on return and partial recovery is estimated to take two to three times as long as the time spent in space. To what extent the rebuilt bone has the desirable architecture and composition is not known. Dr. Lang is following up the recovery of the International Space Station crewmembers with his up-to-the-minute scanning apparatus, and will soon be able to answer this question.

Until fairly recently, bone recovery was considered almost impossible in patients who had suffered spinal cord injury. However, the Herculean personal effort of Christopher Reeve, the 'Superman' star who was paralyzed in a riding accident, had among other discoveries led to ways of restoring much of his bone density. However, rebuilding the right kind of bone in an adult, in the right proportions, in the right places is a great challenge. It is therefore always better, whenever possible, to find ways of preventing the bone loss in the first place.

In space, where there is no loading and no mechanical strain from activity, both hard cortical bone and spongy trabecular bone are lost. In people with spinal cord injury, about one third of cortical and one half of trabecular bone may have been lost before a new steady state is reached. With aging, however, loss of bone mass in the long bones is compensated by a degree of structural remodeling. This helps to maintain the rigidity of bone against the stresses of twisting and bending. The bone continues to grow in diameter as new bone is deposited on its outer surfaces. This makes it stronger, even though its total mass may be less. This deposit of new bone is three times greater in men than in women, making men's bones even stronger as they get older.

What Can You Do about It?

Many factors are involved in the regulation of bone health, but loading is the primary stimulus. Without gravity and the pulling, pushing, and twisting effects of muscles working against gravity, other factors, such as hormones, are less effective. We do not know exactly how bone perceives loading and translates it into a message to build bone tissue. What we do know is that an intact nervous system is needed. Healthy bone, just like any other organ in the body, depends on a good blood supply and on good nerve connections to the central controller, the brain. Promoting good circulation of blood to the bones may be part of the effectiveness of HRT.

The arteries that supply blood to bone tissue lose their stiffness, and hence their efficiency, in space or during bed-rest or inactivity. Patients with spinal-cord injury are still exposed to gravity and have an intact blood supply, bringing calcium and hormones and other nutrients needed by bone tissue. What is missing, then, and why do these patients lose bone? It is because the loading stimulus of gravity is not sensed or transmitted through the nervous system and spine to the brain. This response is needed to keep arteries and bones healthy.

The Value of Good Nutrition

Good nutrition, along with an active lifestyle, helps to defend bones against the effects of aging. But an adequate and balanced diet for the elderly must take into account reduced appetite, as well as changes in absorption, taste, and chewing problems. Eating too much can be as big a problem as eating too little. Excess weight may be good for bone strength, but it puts a stress on weight-bearing joints in the knees, hips, ankles, and feet. One can do much to prevent further damage to the joints by dropping a few pounds and reducing dietary intake of sugar and other inflammation-causing foods.

• Calcium

Adequate calcium is essential for healthy bones, but most elderly people do not eat enough green leafy vegetables and dairy products (milk, cheese, yogurt, eggs, and so on) to get all the calcium they need. Usually four servings of dairy products a day are needed. Spinach and kale are good fat-free sources of calcium, as are high-fat fish such as salmon and sardines. Sesame seeds and almonds are additional good sources. Adults need 1000–1500 mg of calcium a day. One cup of skimmed milk provides 315 mg, and there are 415 mg in one cup of plain low-fat yogurt. One cup of cooked spinach provides 245 mg, and a cup of kale 95 mg. If you do not or cannot take in enough calcium in your diet, supplements are a viable alternative, although they are not preferred.

Your level of activity affects your capacity to absorb this vital bone-manufacturing material. Only one-third to one-half of their calcium intake is absorbed by astronauts in space or by healthy people in bed-rest for four months. Taking more than the daily requirement has the opposite effect to the one intended, for you absorb less. Taking more than 2,000 mg of calcium a day could increase the risk of kidney stones. For most of us, however, taking calcium supplements with vitamin D as we age is a good precaution. Vitamin D is essential for the absorption of calcium, but so is activity. If you are inactive, not much of what you take by mouth will be absorbed. If you suspect you are prone to bone loss, avoid excessive salt in your diet, do not drink more than two cups of coffee a day, and if you smoke, make a serious effort to stop.

• Vitamin D

Vitamin D is manufactured in the liver, but for it to do so the skin has to be exposed to the ultraviolet rays of the sun. Vitamin D helps the gut to absorb calcium, and without it the bones go spongy and become distorted when given weight to bear. This is why, in the early days of the Industrial Revolution, many workers in England's "dark, Satanic mills," who rarely saw daylight and eked out their existence on poor diets, had the typical bow-legs of sufferers from rickets.

Astronauts, who are shielded from ultraviolet light by their spacecraft, return from space with reduced levels of vitamin D. Their levels return to normal with supplements or once they have been exposed to enough daylight. Some exposure to daylight every day is very important. Fifteen minutes a day is believed to be adequate, but more time outdoors is needed if the sun's ultraviolet rays are filtered by clouds. Remember, though, that spending too long in the sun can be damaging to the skin and could lead to skin cancer.

Vitamin-D deficiency is rare these days in the Western world, thanks to the availability of fresh foods (forming part of a balanced diet) and supplements. Liver, egg yolks, and fish liver oil are rich sources, and many foods are fortified with vitamin D. An 8-oz glass of vitamin D-fortified skimmed milk contains 98 units, and one ounce of pickled herring provides 193 units.

Supplements containing vitamin D are in fairly common use, both to prevent bone loss and to treat osteoporosis. Adults need a total daily dose of 400–800 international units. It is usually available in supplements that contain both calcium and vitamin D in one pill. Elderly people, just like astronauts, can become more deficient in vitamin D—probably because they do not spend enough time outdoors.

On the other hand, too much vitamin D—more than 2,000 units a day—can be toxic. It can cause calcium in the blood to rise to abnormal levels, so it is wise to check the total amount you are taking in, especially if you are taking multivitamins as well as consuming it in your diet and supplements. High doses of vitamin D should be avoided if you are taking calcium channel-blocking drugs or diuretics to control high blood pressure. Check with your physician if in doubt.

• Vitamin K

This vitamin is best known for treating blood-clotting disorders. It is, therefore, not recommended for people on anticoagulants. However, it also plays a role in keeping the bones healthy and is believed to help reduce the risk of osteoporosis. Vitamin K is important for making bone proteins. Some studies have linked it to a lower risk of hip fractures, and it may even cut the calcium loss associated with aging. The recommended dose to bring about these benefits is 60–80µg (one tenth of a milligram) a day, but food sources such as citrus fruits, papaya, strawberries, tomatoes, and potatoes should provide all the body needs. Green leafy vegetables, such as lettuce, broccoli, spinach, and Brussels sprouts, are good sources as well. Large doses of vitamin K (up to 500µg) taken for a long period to treat clotting disorders have not given rise to toxic symptoms. The recommended adult dose that may help prevent osteoporosis is 100µg a day.

• Vitamin C

This vitamin has so many benefits that no body should be without it. One of its most important attributes is that it helps produce collagen, the connective tissue that holds bone tissue together. It is a powerful antioxidant that can be found in all citrus fruits, tomatoes, cranberries, and many vegetables. Vitamin C is very unstable and the kidneys get rid of it so quickly that there is no point in taking large doses in supplement form—any excess is simply wasted. It is much more effective to take many smaller doses or, better yet, to get all the vitamin C you need in your diet.

When humans travel to Mars or the Moon, where the availability of fresh fruit and vegetables will be limited, supplements will become very important. In the days of sailing ships, when the dietary virtues of vitamins and the fruit and vegetables that contained them were undreamed of, anybody who undertook a long journey by sea ran a high risk of scurvy. This unlovely disease, which causes internal bleeding and loosens the gums so that the teeth fall out, afflicted the seventeenth-century *Mayflower* pilgrims.

• Minerals

Apart from the all-important calcium, phosphorus is another mineral that is needed to build bones. It is found in dairy products, such as yogurt, eggs, and cheese, and in many other foods, including nuts, meat, and fish. In fact, it is so widely available that you are more likely to have an excess of this mineral rather than a deficiency. But too much is not good either. Drinking soda pop, for instance, can lead to an overabundance of phosphorus, which, together with a low calcium intake, has been blamed for deficiencies in bone building.

Magnesium, copper, and chromium are needed by the body only in minute amounts and are known as trace elements. They too are critical for healthy bone. They are found in green vegetables and nuts and play a part in increasing bone density and strength. The bottom line is that a diet rich in fresh fruits and vegetables, dairy products, nuts, and fish should provide all the vitamins and minerals that are needed. If for some reason this is not possible, supplements will have to do but monitoring doses is important.

Steroids and Other Hormones
• Sex Steroids: Hormone Replacement Therapy

Estrogen, administered in hormone replacement therapy (HRT), has probably been the most widely used drug for preventing menopause-associated bone loss. It is available in pills or as a patch. It comes either as 17-B-Estradiol, the natural human hormone, or as estrogens extracted from the urine of pregnant mares and sold under the trade names of Premarin or Provera. In women who have not had a hysterectomy, estrogens are always given with progesterone to prevent cancer of the uterus.

Once touted as the answer to all postmenopausal ills, estrogen is now being reevaluated. It clearly reduces bone loss in women who lose a lot of bone going through the menopause, but its usefulness appears to be limited in its duration. Bone loss resumes at the faster rate after two or three years even with the continued use of estrogen. Though a dwindling natural supply of estrogen is a major factor, it does not appear to be the sole cause of bone loss or osteoporosis after the menopause.

One much-anticipated benefit from HRT was the prevention of cardiovascular disease, the likelihood of which increases in women after menopause. However, in a fifteen-year study of 161,000 women undertaken by the National Institutes of Health, those taking Premarin actually showed a higher incidence of cardiovascular disease. This was sufficiently worrying for that portion of the study to be terminated five years early. In 2004, another segment of this study in women taking estrogen after hysterectomies was terminated for the same reason. A higher incidence of breast cancer has also been found in another portion of this same study, as well as in studies in a much larger number of women in England. As a result of these side effects, there has been a massive reaction against all forms of HRT

It was once assumed that all changes after menopause were due to the reduction of estrogen and that HRT would prevent them. But a study comparing women who had never taken estrogen with those who stopped HRT even after taking it for ten years showed no difference either in the density of their bones or in the number of fractures they suffered. HRT does prevent some of the symptoms of menopause, such as hot flashes. It makes skin plumper and more elastic. Estrogen is a potent antioxidant, fighting off some of the aging effects of free radicals. But there is now some uncertainty as to whether it brings other benefits once claimed—such as an improved memory or protection against Alzheimer's disease.

One aspect that has not been explored is that of dosage. When a doctor says, "I am giving you the lowest possible dose," what he or she really means is "the lowest dose the manufacturer produces." It is not unlikely that much lower doses than those commercially available in tablets may be effective in preventing unpleasant hot flashes and even protecting bone, without the undesirable side effects such as blood clots. Lower amounts of estrogen-like substances can also be found in soy products.

Genetic predisposition is an important factor in post-menopausal bone loss and in the development of osteoporosis. It also influences the response to estrogen and to other drugs. Small, light-skinned women with a genetic predisposition to osteoporosis benefit most from HRT. However, although estrogen provides many benefits, let us not forget that today's active over-eighty-year-olds, especially the centenarians, somehow managed without ever taking HRT. They may be genetically resistant to osteoporosis or have led very active lives.

• Sex Steroids: Testosterone

Because production of the male sex hormone, testosterone, decreases only gradually with age—it falls by about 1% a year after age forty—its effects on bone have not been a matter of great concern. Bone loss in men becomes more evident in their mid-seventies. However, testosterone is necessary for the growth and maintenance of bones. Only one man in five between the ages of sixty and eighty has a lower level of testosterone than is normal for his age, so lack of the hormone is not a widespread problem. In one study, testosterone replacement was given over a three-year period to men over seventy, and a modest increase in bone mineral density was achieved.

Testosterone can be administered in patches, just like estrogen, but in our present state of knowledge, the disadvantages of using it to treat older men for bone loss are greater than its benefits. It can stimulate the growth of prostate tissue, adding to the risk of prostate cancer. It can increase the possibility of cardio-vascular disease, cause sleep apnea—the intermittent cessation of breathing during sleep—lead to fluid retention, and cause depression.

• Corticosteroids

Cortisol (hydrocortisone) is a steroid made by the adrenal gland. Even more powerful synthetic relatives, such as prednisolone or betamethasone, are also available. Corticosteroids are mostly used as a last resort in a variety of inflammation conditions and have proven miraculously effective. But they also have serious side effects.

People with allergic conditions or with severe joint inflammation, such as bursitis (tennis elbow), are sometimes treated with these steroids. They are also found in some over-the-counter creams used to soothe itching and the kind of severe skin inflammation that one may experience as a reaction to poison ivy.

These steroids are potent in breaking down collagen not only in bone but in muscle, joints, tendons, ligaments, and skin as well. They have this effect whether taken orally, by local injection, or even when applied externally as a cream. Injected into painful joints, they give almost instant relief that lasts for several months. However, frequent use will break down the collagen in the area and weaken tendons and ligaments, potentially causing long-term problems. They should not be used more than twice a year. The overuse of steroid creams can cause visible thinning of the skin. Treatment with corticosteroids is only available by prescription and should be resorted to with special caution in the case of elderly people and patients who have already suffered significant bone loss.

• Calcitonin

This is another hormone that regulates bone formation which has potential benefits. But it is not for everybody. Calcitonin, produced by the thyroid gland, prevents osteoclasts from promoting bone loss, but also increases the loss of calcium by the kidneys. It is therefore used only in special cases. It has been used successfully in unusual circumstances, such as to reduce back pain in women who are at least five years past the menopause and suffer from fractured vertebrae. It is injected or given as a nasal spray.

Drugs

Drug companies have placed a heavy emphasis on developing non-hormonal drugs that target bone loss to meet the needs of the ballooning older population in the U.S.

• Bisphosphonates

Chemicals called bisphosphonates, taken in pill form or by injection, concentrate in bone and inhibit bone loss by switching off osteoclasts and reducing their numbers. Two of them, alendronate (trade name Fosamax) and risedronate (trade name Actonel) are currently used to treat patients suffering from osteoporosis. Unfortunately, they are sometimes prescribed as a preventive measure for people who begin to show bone density that is lower than what is considered normal for their age group when perhaps other measures have not been exhausted.

An unpleasant aspect of taking these drugs is the need to ensure absorption and prevent serious stomach irritation. Users must take the pills on an empty stomach with a full glass of water then remain upright for at least thirty minutes. Benefits reported have been 3 to 5% increased bone density and a 50% lower risk of bone fractures compared with those who took nothing. It is too early to say what the side effects of their long-term use may be. New bisphosphonates that are effective for one year after a single injection will soon be available.

• Raloxifene

Raloxifene (trade name Evista) belongs to a class of drugs known as SERMs (Selective Estrogen Receptor Modulators), which act like estrogen in some ways but not in all. For instance, Raloxifene does not prevent hot flashes, nor does it stop the formation of blood clots in leg veins, a condition that afflicts some women on HRT. However, like estrogen, it retards bone loss. And it lowers cholesterol without increasing the risk of breast or uterine cancer. In fact, its beneficial action on bone was discovered when it was used as a possible treatment for breast cancer. In clinical trials on post-menopausal women, it increased bone density by 3 to 4% and reduced by 40% the risk of fractures of the vertebrae.

• Strontium Ranelate

An old drug may be the new thing in treating osteoporosis. Strontium is an element that is very closely related to calcium. It was widely used in the fifties to help build bones, until it fell out of favor over concerns that high doses interfered with vitamin-D production. However, French researchers recently found that a low dose of strontium ranelate, a new version of the drug, taken with vitamin D and calcium supplements, cut spinal fractures by 41% over three years in women with osteoporosis. It also increased bone density by 14% by making new bone tissue grow, whereas bisphosphonates like Fosamax only harden existing bone. Clinical trials are ongoing.

• Osteoprotegerin

Scientists at the biotechnology company Amgen have identified a protein called osteoprotegerin, which prevents the formation and activation of the osteoclasts that break down bone tissue. This means it has the potential to stave off excessive bone loss, or osteoporosis. Other groups joined the search, and a class of regulatory proteins is being discovered that point the way to new ways of preserving bone mass.

In clinical tests, a single dose of osteoprotegerin, given by injection to postmenopausal women, slowed down the rate of bone loss for weeks after treatment. These are the early stages for what could be a promising line of treatment for osteoporosis, and especially for bone loss due to cancer. The story is not yet complete, but every day brings us closer to understanding how to protect our bones.

• Doxycycline

We may not associate periodontal disease or gum disease with our bones, but this is probably the most common bone disease. Bacteria accumulate in the space between the gum and the neck of the tooth, leading to a buildup of dental plaque—a film of bacteria, saliva, mucus, and food residues. The bacterial infection causes inflammation of gum tissue and increases the activity of the enzymes that break down collagen in the bony tissue of teeth.

The antibiotic doxycycline (trade name Periostat), given in doses so small (25 mg) that they have no antibiotic activity, has proven very effective in treating gum disease. It is reported to act by preventing an increase in the activity of collagenase, the enzyme that breaks down collagen. Any drug that prevents the breakdown of collagen by collagenase has broad therapeutic value. Doxycycline has been going through tests at the University of Nebraska for possible beneficial effects on bone. It is possible that it may also be useful in reducing the collagen loss in joints that is associated with arthritis.

• Statins

For some time, people have been taking the class of drugs known as statins (trade names Lipitor and Zocor) to lower their blood cholesterol and reduce the risk of heart attacks. Doctors noticed by chance that those taking them had stronger bones. Researchers followed up this observation and noted an increased rate of bone formation and a reduced risk of fractures in patients taking statins. Properly controlled clinical trials are now pointing the way to important benefits.

• Anti-inflammatory Drugs

Because pain and inflammation are the primary symptoms of joint injuries and arthritis, anti-inflammatory drugs were first given for the relief of pain. Acetaminophen (trade name Tylenol) is only mildly effective for this purpose. Ibuprofen (trade names Advil and Motrin) and naproxen (trade name Aleve) are more effective but can cause stomach irritation. The newer class of COX-2 inhibitor chemicals (trade names Vioxx and Celebrex) reduce inflammation and though they do not produce stomach ulcers and bleeding, they do increase the risk of heart attacks and strokes.

Supplements
• Fluoride

Commonly added to water supplies to prevent tooth decay, fluoride has been shown to increase the mineral density of spinal bone. In a forty-two-month study, fluoride reduced by 68% the risk of a second vertebral fracture in eighty-five post-menopausal women older than sixty-five who had already suffered one vertebral fracture. The fluoride was given in a slow-release form that has not yet been approved by the U.S. Food and Drug Administration.

• Glucosamine and Chondroitin

Physical wear and tear of joints, caused by running or jogging on hard surfaces, can cause osteoarthritis, an inflammation of the joints caused by the degeneration of collagen in its cartilage lining. Cartilage is also a casualty of aging, and its loss makes knees, hips, and ankles very tender and sore, because when the cartilage goes, bone rubs against bone. Recent new approaches to treating the loss of collagen have come from an unlikely source, the racetrack. Glucosamine and chondroitin are found in the protein of bone, skin, and joint cells. For some time, they have been given in large doses to racehorses suffering joint injuries. They have also been applied in gels to accelerate the healing of wounds, becoming part of the tissue as it heals.

Glucosamine and chondroitin work together to block the action of enzymes that destroy collagen and cartilage. They provide relief to aching joints in professional football players, fitness enthusiasts, surgeons, and others who spend a lot of their time on their feet. Much of the information about their positive effects on humans has been anecdotal. However, studies in France, Portugal, and Italy found that daily doses of 1,500 mg glucosamine and 1,200 mg chondroitin reduced symptoms of arthritis by 73% after four to six weeks. It is recommended that this dose, ideal for a 120–200 lb person, should be taken for eight weeks and reduced after that to 500–1,000 mg glucosamine and 400–800 mg chondroitin per day, depending on the level of relief.

An extensive study of the value of these substances as treatments for arthritis, both alone and together, is underway, sponsored by the National Institutes of Health. It is generally estimated that at least one-third of patients with arthritis get pain relief with these supplements. Hip and knee joints seem to benefit most. There are no known side effects.

Exercise

Using common sense is crucial when exercising. Jogging may be excellent for your heart and bones, yet it may not do your knees and hips much good. An orthopedic surgeon I know says he has fifty-year-olds coming to his office who are aerobically fit enough to live to ninety, but whose joints are already those of a ninety-year-old. Yet for more than seventeen years, Jim Fries at Stanford University in California studied more than 500 joggers and over 400 couch potatoes and found that only 5% of his runners suffered joint problems compared with 20% of the sedentary group. Wear and tear, injury, worn-out shoes, and running on hard surfaces were more to blame than the actual running.

Proper exercise, with the proper footwear and on resilient surfaces, reduces joint pain and improves function. Some exercises improve flexibility of the joints, some build bone mass, and others, such as weight training and resistance exercises, strengthen the muscles that support the joints.

• Use the Stairs

Climbing the stairs is a very effective comprehensive exercise. It stimulates weight-bearing muscles and joints as well as the heart. Walking down stairs provides impact loading to bone with each step and helps coordination—benefits that are only partially achieved on stair-master exercise equipment. Whatever your age, "never take an elevator unless it is more than six floors" is a worthy aim.

• Wearing Weights

Put weights around your waist to increase your body loading when you walk. Make sure it is evenly distributed. Bear in mind that obese people have stronger bones because of the extra weight they carry. It also feels great when you take the weights off at the end of your walk! Medium- and long-distance runners often train with weights on their backs so as to improve their performance during the actual race.

• Impact-loading, Weight-bearing Exercises

Weight bearing, or loading, is the critical factor in maintaining bone mass and density. In older people, even short periods of standing may help reduce the risk of fracture. Even those who are unable to stand could benefit from being passively tilted up on a tilt table or bed; also, wearing a supporting harness to provide some downward load may help in reducing the risk of fracture.

Walking, running, going down the stairs, and weight training are all impact-loading, weight-bearing exercises. Bicycling and swimming involve less impact and much less weight-bearing force. This does not mean that they do not produce some benefit, but they are not the best activity for bones. A study of tennis players showed that the bones of their dominant arm were markedly thicker and stronger than those of the other arm. If bone is to be strengthened and new bone is to be built by exercise, the mechanical stress placed on it by an activity must go beyond the level to which it has become accustomed.

Research has shown that to stimulate new bone formation, you need short periods of intense loading rather than long-term, routine, constant loading. However, to maintain bone density, you need sustained loading, so it pays to vary the kind of exercise you take.

Just as with muscle, bone mass reverts to pre-exercise levels when weight-bearing exercise is discontinued. A recent study at Oregon State University on twenty-nine pre-menopausal women aged thirty-five to forty found that their bone density increased after twelve months of impact and resistance training but that all the benefits were lost after only six months of "detraining." The exercises in this study, designed to stimulate hip-bone density, were strenuous. Participants trained three times a week, doing nine sets of ten to twelve jumping exercises, such as jumping jacks. Also included were nine sets of ten to twelve squats and lunges. The challenge was upped as time progressed, and the women were asked to wear weighted vests. They gained 2.5 to 2.7% density in their thigh-bones. The study showed that it is easier to lose bone by being inactive than to gain new bone by loading. Preventing bone loss in the first place is so important. But reversing bone loss is possible.

David Upton, speaking for the American Council on Exercise, advises weight training for all adults at least twice a week, allowing time between sessions for the body to recover. It is important to "surprise" bone by interspersing weight training with impact activities, such as jumping, stepping up or down, walking, gymnastics, or playing volleyball.

As with muscle, but even more so with bone, the message is not to put off taking up exercise, whatever your age.

My healthy volunteers who were confined to bed could regain bone density after they resumed weight-bearing activity. But people who are permanently bedridden and can never resume weight-bearing activities do not regain lost bone density, although stress on bones from any muscular activity (even in bed) can be beneficial. But experience in space, without gravity, shows that as much as four hours a day of vigorous exercise is of limited value without the loading provided by the body's weight in gravity. In fact, Sue Schneider at the University of New Mexico and her colleagues in Houston concluded that astronauts performing resistive exercise in space will require much greater forces than Earth's 1G to provide a sufficient stimulus to maintain bone and muscle mass.

Physical Interventions

Physical interventions for protecting arthritic joints can be as simple as getting shock-absorbing footwear, wearing wedge-shaped insoles to redistribute weight, taping the knees, wearing a knee brace, or using a cane or walker for support. Knee surgery to remove loose pieces of bone or cartilage, or to smooth rough bone surfaces in the joint, will also help relieve pain. As a last resort, surgery to replace hip, knee, or shoulder joints can restore most of their functions and eliminate pain.

Interventions to prevent bone loss or build new bone are of a different nature. Several different approaches have been tried. Most are still experimental, but some show promise. They include magnetic stimulation, electrical stimulation of supporting muscles, vibration, and increased loading by means of hypergravity on a centrifuge. The pattern, frequency, and magnitude of the gravity stimulus provided by these interventions are crucial. So little is known about these optimal characteristics that an approach is often abandoned after a few trials though it may show some promise.

• Magnetic Stimulation

Thirty to thirty-five years ago, there was a great deal of interest in surrounding a broken arm or leg with a magnetic coil to accelerate repair. Although the research at first looked very promising, it was never fully substantiated and the tests were abandoned.

• Electrical Muscle Stimulation (EMS)

The effect of EMS on bone is indirect. It works by strengthening the contractions of supporting muscles. EMS of the legs was tried in patients paralyzed from injury to the spinal cord. Although muscle benefits were greater than those to bone, the rate of bone loss was less than would otherwise have been expected. EMS may not stop or reverse bone loss, but slowing down the rate of bone loss is in itself a very positive result. Where it can be done, EMS with some physical training appears to be highly beneficial in preventing muscle atrophy, maintaining aerobic capacity, and even improving gait.

• Vibration

Vigorous exercise and EMS are believed to increase bone mass because of the high-magnitude, low-frequency strain muscles put on bone. The muscle contractions are strong but not too fast. Vibration, by contrast, provides high-frequency, low-intensity strain: the stimulus is very frequent but mild. Clinton Rubin at State University of New York, in Stony Brook, N.Y., believes that this is the kind of stimulus that bone senses when loaded. He found that the kind of strain that muscles continuously place on bones while a person is sitting or standing is close to the oscillations provided by vibration and are important in preserving bone mass. It therefore has the added advantage of improving muscle performance. He believes these oscillations "trick" the body into thinking it is receiving a load-bearing strain, and the bones get stiffer and stronger.

Standing on Rubin's vibrating platform for as little as ten minutes improves both the quality and quantity of bone. The vibrating platform provides barely perceptible oscillations. Rubin tested a menagerie of mice, rats, turkeys, sheep, and humans on his vibrating platform with positive results. In a one-year study, sheep standing on the platform for twenty minutes a day showed a 34% increase in trabecular bone and a 26% increase in bone strength. Studies with post-menopausal women standing on his vibrating platform have also been positive.

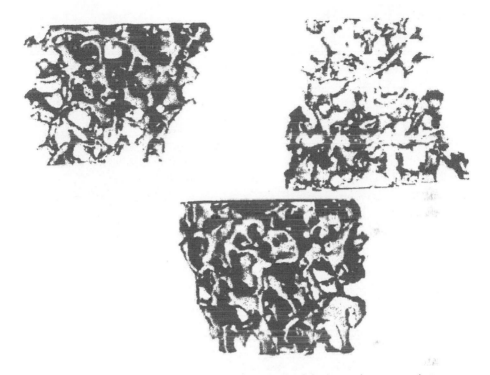

Effect of Vibration on bone loss and repair: Top left picture shows normal
bone; top right picture shows the bone loss associated with unloading, such
as inactivity or living in space. (Note more white spaces where bone was
lost.) Bottom picture is from unloaded bone treated with vibration therapy.
Looks darker more dense, with fewer white spaces.
(Rubin et al., NASA archive)

Rubin now hopes to test his platform on astronauts in space. But if it is
expected to work in space it should also benefit persons with spinal cord injury
who cannot sense their body's load. It may also provide a promising way of
increasing bone mass and diminishing the risk of fractures in those who are bedridden or have difficulty standing. This vibrating platform is not yet commercially available.

• Hypergravity

The importance of gravity's loading effect on bone was demonstrated by scientists in Perth, Australia. Fighter pilots performing aerial combat maneuvers experience high stress loads on their vertebrae. As the head-to-toe G-force increases,
so does the loading on the spine and pelvis. Fiona Naumann at the Edith Cowan

University, in Perth, and her colleagues monitored the bone response of a group of young Royal Australian Air Force fighter pilots on a twelve-month high-performance flight-training course. G-forces generated during their advanced aerobatic maneuvers averaged around three to four times Earth's gravity. At the end of the training period, the pilots had an 11% increase in bone-mineral density in the thoracic spine (the upper part of the spinal column) and a 5% increase in the density of the pelvic bones.

I am not, of course, suggesting putting the elderly through aerobatic maneuvers to increase their bone density or giving them rides on roller coasters to give them a dose of hypergravity. But various acceleration devices (such as centrifuges) exist, and they could provide patients with short, graded exposure to increased gravity loads. Such hypergravity treatment could be targeted at specific areas and might be especially useful for patients who cannot support themselves or are injured. In space, where there is minimal gravity, bone fractures take longer to heal. Logically, then, one might hope that hypergravity treatment would accelerate the healing process. This theory remains to be tested, but as the evidence accumulates, the therapeutic usefulness of hypergravity, gravity treatment on a centrifuge, will surely come into its own.

The Varied Approach

Minimizing bone loss and protecting joints from wear and tear are essential goals for anybody concerned about healthy and active aging. But there is no magic bullet. No single treatment is the absolute answer—but preserving collagen is crucial. A balanced combination of treatments is more likely to be effective.

As in everything else, good genes are an asset. They determine who is most likely to suffer bone fractures and how bones will respond to drugs or other treatments. Fundamental ingredients for the building and maintenance of healthy bones include loading—both by gravity and through weight-bearing, impact-loading activities—and proper nutrition. Physical interventions are always preferable before resorting to drugs. Bone loss can be stopped, and it can be reversed.

3

Flexing Muscle

o o o o o o o o o o o o o o o o o o o o o o o o o o o o o o o o o

Muscles come and go; flab lasts.

—*Bill Vaughan, 1915–1977*

"Chicken Legs!"

That's how fellow astronauts greeted Pete Conrad and the other *Gemini V* crewmember returning from space in 1965, even though Conrad tried to show off his fitness by doing push-ups on the ship's flight deck. In space, muscles that work against gravity are no longer needed or used. They become the first targets of unloading—that is, they shed the burden of carrying around the body's weight.

The same thing happens if you stay off your feet for a long time. Unloading may seem like a kind of holiday for these muscles, but it is not a good thing. It leads to a shrinking of mass, and with this comes a loss in strength and endurance. Most affected are leg muscles and those that support the hips, spine, and head. Muscles work by contracting, either to stretch out limbs (the extensors) or to pull limbs closer together (the flexors). Flexor muscles, such as the biceps, are less affected in space, because they continue to be used. All the work carried out by astronauts is done with their arms—pushing and pulling items of equipment from their racks, prying things open, or doing strenuous jobs outside the spacecraft using their pressurized gloves.

Fighting the Flab

The Gemini astronauts came back skinny legged, but with Larry De Lucas, returning in 1992 from just a few days in space on *STS-50*, it was the arms that were most visibly affected. Describing his horror at their flabbiness, he said they looked like "those of an old lady." He was just forty-two. Women especially can identify with Larry's dismay at the condition of his arms. Nothing hits home quite as hard as watching with apprehension as your underarms begin to hang and jiggle—a powerful hint that the time has come to donate your sleeveless dresses to a good cause.

Underarm muscles get flabby as we age, even though we are in gravity all the time. This happens because we quit doing certain kinds of work, such as raising heavy objects above our heads, and so no longer target gravity towards these muscles. Men's underarm muscles stay firm longer, but they are not exempt from such changes either. Is there something we can do about it? Larry's arms got back to their firm state with some tailored weight training during his rehabilitation. There is no reason why ours cannot.

"But," you may say, "I walk three miles three times a week and I go to my aerobics class once a week, and I still cannot seem to prevent this flab." Exercising regularly is commendable, and you should continue doing it. But the type of exercise you are doing may not be making too many demands on muscles that are specifically designed to support weight and to work against gravity, those that protect us from falling. When was the last time you used gravity to target the muscle groups that support your body's weight? When did you last do push-ups, pull-ups, or some other kind of weight lifting? Perhaps you did not think of pushing up or pulling up the weight of your body as weight lifting.

How the System Works

Muscle is second to the brain in its importance to a healthy body and serves many functions. Skeletal muscle supports and protects the skeleton. It is also the body's factory, making protein and burning carbohydrates to generate energy. Heart muscle is the body's pump, sending blood to the rest of the body. Smooth muscle makes up the tubes that transport blood, food, urine, eggs, or sperm to hollow-muscle organs such as the stomach, intestines, bladder, and uterus. This chapter will focus on skeletal muscle only.

Why Athletes Need to Warm Up

Skeletal muscles work in pairs, so that as one contracts, moving one of the many levers in the skeleton, its partner relaxes. This is why sprinters always need to warm up thoroughly before the start of a race. If the hamstring muscles at the back of the thigh cannot relax quickly enough to keep pace with the contractions of the powerful muscles at the front of the thigh, there is a high risk that they will tear.

The muscles that support the skeleton are made up of bundles of long, thin fibers embedded in collagen, the same fibrous protein that is also found in bones, joints, tendons, and the skin. The bundles consist of dark and light sections, depending on the distribution of two proteins, actin and myosin. When the muscle contracts to perform work of any kind, the lighter actin sections slide between the myosin sections. They combine to form actomyosin, making the muscle thicker and shorter. Muscle relaxation results when actin and myosin are returned to their original separate states.

There are fast-twitch and slow-twitch skeletal muscles. Contraction is more rapid in pale muscle fibers ("fast-twitch") than in the darker fibers ("slow-twitch"). Pale fibers are predominant in muscles like the biceps and the thigh muscles, which are used when a fast reaction is essential. They are mostly involved in walking, running, bicycling, swimming, and skating. Dark fibers predominate in slow-twitch muscles, such as those supporting the spine or those such as the soleus in the calf of the leg, which need to contract steadily for hours at a time to hold up the body. If they are underused they are much more difficult to maintain or restore than fast-twitch muscles.

How strong a person is depends on the number and cross-sectional area of his or her muscle fibers. The larger the muscle, the more weight it can carry, and the more weight it carries, the bigger the muscle gets. If there is no weight to carry, as in space, or if you avoid carrying weight by cutting down on physical activity, muscles will atrophy.

When we think of youth we think of firm, strong bodies. This is the ideal self-image at any age, but apart from looks, keeping your muscles strong is essential to living an independent life. Being able to step up without fear onto a bus can make the difference between getting about or not venturing out of the house. Being able to carry your grandchild safely may make the difference between pleasure and feeling worthless. Going up or down three steps carrying two bags of groceries may seem like an impossible task to some. Kneeling to put away dishes in the cabinets under the kitchen counter and standing up without help or a groan can become a challenge.

When I give talks and see that the audience has slumped nicely into their chairs, I ask them to jump up without using their arms or hands. I am constantly amazed at how many under the age of fifty-five are unable to jump to their feet from a sitting position without grasping the chair. But this does not have to be the fate of us all as we pass fifty.

The Muscle Factory

Most people think of skeletal muscle as important only for support, movement, strength, and looks. Few are aware that one of the major roles of muscle is to act as the body's factory. It is essential for synthesizing protein, a necessary step towards building lean body mass. Several hormones act on muscle in the all-important process of keeping it healthy. The hormone insulin, from the pancreas, attaches to muscle cells to promote the transport of glucose from the bloodstream into the cells. Glucose is then used as fuel to generate energy. The amount of muscle, its mass, then becomes very important in determining how much glucose is burnt and how much energy can be generated.

The stress hormone, cortisol (hydrocortisone), is catabolic, a technical term meaning that it breaks down protein. When we feel stressed, greater amounts of cortisol are produced. This has a dramatic effect, causing the loss of muscle and bone mass. The sex steroid, testosterone, on the other hand, is anabolic, meaning that it promotes the manufacture of protein and builds up muscle. Testosterone and other anabolic steroids have gained great popularity in the muscle-building community. We do not know exactly why, but without gravity, anabolic steroids do not do their job as well, whereas catabolic steroids become even more destructive.

Growth hormone also plays an important role in helping the muscles to manufacture protein. It is produced by the pituitary gland at the base of the brain and secreted in pulses, mostly during the first few hours of sleep or in response to exercise. Sound sleep and regular exercise are therefore the best ways to keep growth-hormone levels up. This hormone, essential for the growth of cells in bones, muscle, and organs, is particularly important for normal development in children. Its production peaks at adolescence.

The Importance of Muscle in Supporting the Body

You may have a good sense of balance and your heart and circulation may be in good condition, but you may still fall because your leg muscles have become too weak to support your weight. Skeletal muscles are responsible for body posture, but also for movement and physical work. They form 40% of body mass in men and about 25% in women. A group of muscles that counteract the pull of gravity have developed over the course of human evolution. These muscles are concentrated in the lower back, neck, abdomen, and legs. Their function is to allow erect posture, supporting the head over the spinal column and centering the body over the pelvis and legs. The center of gravity in a healthy body is in the mid-pelvis. This shifts to the middle of the back and lower chest on lying down.

What Can Go Wrong?

Growth of muscle peaks at about age twenty to thirty. The muscle mass you can expect forty or fifty years later depends on two factors: the maximum mass achieved in your twenties and the rate at which it is lost after that. Both of these factors vary among individuals. Some start losing muscle earlier than others. The average rate of muscle loss after reaching maximum mass is about 0.5–1% per year. Muscle atrophy is generally not viewed as a disease, although if it goes too far it can affect the ability to live an independent life.

Sarcopenia, Greek for "short on flesh," means muscle wasting. It occurs when catabolism, the breakdown of protein, exceeds anabolism, or protein build up. In general, catabolism increases and anabolism decreases with age, stress, and inactivity. Patients with AIDS, osteoporosis, or depression also show such serious muscle wasting. It is a feature of advanced aging. Even in seniors who take regular exercise and keep in good health and fitness, there may be a sudden unexplained onset of sarcopenia, which can be very hard to reverse.

Several studies underscore the importance of viewing sarcopenia as a public-health problem. For instance, in1999, the Mayo Clinic, in Rochester, Minnesota, ran a random sample study of the local population, and a 1998 study in New Mexico used both Hispanics and non-Hispanics. Both surveys confirmed that lean body mass progressively decreases after age twenty at the same rate in men and women.

How Spaceflight Weakens Muscles

We have learned much from space about how muscles change if they are relieved of the burden of carrying around the body's weight. They get smaller and weaker. They are metabolically less efficient and generate less energy. Their properties can change from slow-twitch to fast-twitch, since gravity-countering slow-twitch muscles are no longer needed in space. Experiments in space have confirmed that the reductions in the mass, force of contraction, endurance, and function of muscles are due to an immediate decrease in the rate of protein synthesis. As the flight goes on, this decrease in available protein is compounded by the breakdown and degradation of whatever protein remains.

Muscles that support the spine are stretched as astronauts get taller in space-flight without the compressing influence of Earth's gravity. However, after landing, back pain is quite common, for the return to gravity compresses the vertebrae and the weakened muscles are in no condition to provide the required support.

Reduced muscle protein means less endurance of muscles like the soleus in the back of the leg, which normally respond to gravity and support the body's weight. Endurance, or the ability to resist fatigue, is measured by how long an electrically stimulated muscle can hold a contraction before quitting. As much as a 40% decrease in endurance has been measured in rats after as little as fourteen days in space.

The ability of muscle metabolism to provide energy is also affected when gravity is not present. The energy needed for a sustained contraction results from the breakdown of the glucose and glycogen carbohydrates stored in muscle interacting with oxygen. If these are not available, the body may turn to fatty acids as a source of energy. However, the muscle fibers have a lower capacity to combine oxygen with fatty acids, so less energy is produced using this source.

The Consequences of Inactivity

Visualize a weightlifter who has stopped exercising. What you see is flab, because fat moves in to replace the lost muscle. It is not only esthetically less appealing, but the muscle factory becomes less productive. Over the past ten years, a number of surveys and reports have documented the relationship between activity and present-day killer diseases such as high blood pressure, osteoporosis, diabetes, and depression. Frank Booth and his colleagues at the University of Missouri have calculated that "physical inactivity potentiates at least seventeen unhealthy conditions at the cost of nearly $1 trillion a year."

It has been known for some time that glucose uptake by muscle is reduced in people suffering from diabetes. They therefore require more insulin to transport the required amount of glucose to the muscles. Even in healthy non-diabetics, inactivity makes muscle more resistant to the action of insulin, so that more insulin is required to produce the same effect. Exercise, on the other hand, increases the sensitivity of muscle to insulin. It is now known that exercise stimulates the mechanism in the muscle cell membranes that transports glucose into the cell.

Healthy volunteers in bed-rest for as little as seven days show a much larger and longer increase in their blood-sugar levels after drinking a sugary drink than they did when they were up and about. This test, known as the glucose-tolerance test (GTT), is widely used to detect diabetes, so bed-rest was resulting in volunteers having a glucose profile like that of a diabetic. But unlike diabetics, these volunteers had no problem secreting insulin. In fact, they poured out more insulin as well. However, this did not help reduce the blood sugar. The problem was that the inactivity in bed-rest was preventing the muscle from taking up the glucose. The reverse was found in 1963, when the highly fit members of a Norwegian ski patrol were given a GTT. Hardly any increase in blood sugar was seen after drinking all that sugar.

Complaints of generalized muscle aches and feelings of tiredness are common even in healthy people who stay in bed for as little as twenty-four hours. People who are inactive commonly suffer from backache, just as astronauts do after being in space. But there are also complaints from them about pain in the neck, arms, and legs. A change in body position in bed sometimes temporarily relieves these aches, though for some people the very act of turning over can be painful.

Bad Habits That Can Cause Back Pain

Bad posture when sitting or standing will affect the body's natural center of gravity. Try not to get into the habit of slouching or carrying a weight, such as a child, a briefcase, a computer, or even a large handbag, regularly to one side. Shifting the body's center of gravity forces muscles other than the gravity-countering muscles to assume important support roles for the head, shoulders, and back, and this is not what they were designed for. Asking a muscle to contract when it has not worked for a while can send that muscle into a painful spasm—a sudden seizing up.

Most back problems result from such a muscle spasm pulling on the sciatic nerve, or sagging abdominal muscles and bad posture pulling the unsupported spine forward. Lucky are those who have never experienced back pain at some time in their lives. It is estimated that at least half the U.S. population at any one time suffers from bad pain. It is estimated that it costs the nation $28 billion a year in healthcare costs alone, not to mention work absenteeism and plain old misery.

The Way We Use Muscle Matters

One of the most striking changes that happen to muscles in space is that the fibers of muscles that support posture convert from slow-twitch to fast-twitch. This can happen after just one week in space. Inactivity can cause this shift as well, but it happens more slowly.

Men aged thirty to fifty returning from fourteen days in space, or after thirty days in bed, show reductions in their muscle fibers that are remarkably similar to those in men over the age of seventy here on Earth. Biopsies of the thigh muscle (the *vastus lateralis*, which is composed mostly of fast-twitch fibers) show that in all three groups there are fewer and smaller fibers, with less capacity to generate aerobic energy. The fibers also look structurally disorganized, unlike the neat parallel bundles found in healthy, active muscle.

Even immobilization in a cast produces similar results. When a twenty-two-year-old cross-country skier in Colorado had his leg put in a cast for a torn knee ligament, the total volume of the leg muscles decreased. However, the proportion of fast-twitch fibers, those used to walk and ski, fell from 80% at the time of surgery to 57% after just one month in the cast.

The way we use or do not use muscles determines their type. Crossing over nerves that normally supply fast-twitch muscle and connecting them surgically to slow-twitch muscle can change the fiber type. Slow-twitch muscle can be converted to fast-twitch by reconnecting the nerve supply. The reverse is also true. This is because muscle responds to the pattern of electrical stimulation that comes down the nerve. One type of muscle fiber can also be changed to the other by frequent electrical stimulation over long periods of time.

The knowledge that muscle fibers can be changed by the type of electrical or nerve impulse they receive is now used in the rehabilitation of spinal-cord injuries, sports injuries, muscular dystrophy, and deterioration through aging. One day it may be used to prevent muscle atrophy in astronauts on their way to Mars.

A 'Holiday' from Gravity Makes Muscle Injury More Likely

Biopsies in the vastus lateralis of men over seventy also show 23% fewer muscle fibers than in twenty-five to thirty-year-olds. These fibers are also less able to develop new nerve connections if they are damaged. Fat and connective tissue move in to replace the damaged fibers. Being in space has a similar effect, making muscle fibers more susceptible to injury and slower to heal. A fair number of astronauts, eager to get back to full fitness, have had reason to regret going out jogging too soon after their return from space. They end up with torn muscles or ligaments in their legs, which needed longer to re-attune themselves to gravity. Such muscle damage occurs not while they are in space but only after landing.

Muscle Health as We Grow Older

Gradual and progressive inactivity as one gets older can, over years, produce many of the symptoms that total bed-rest or a flight in space will bring about in weeks or months. The muscle weakness and soreness, fatigue, and faulty coordination that astronauts experience after spaceflight are just like the changes seen in bed-ridden patients when they get up or in many elderly people after unaccustomed exertion.

In spaceflights of up to six months, astronauts lose muscle mass at an average rate of 0.5–1% per week, compared to a loss of 0.5–1% per year on Earth. This telescoping of the effects of unloading on both muscle and bone is a valuable tool in understanding the much more gradual changes that come with aging.

The "Gravity Gene"

Advances in understanding muscle responses to gravity have led to the identification of a gene related to myosin that has been referred to as the "gravity gene," because it passes instructions to the body only in the presence of gravity. A similar gene related to actin, which together with myosin makes up muscle fiber, has also been identified.

There is a loss of motor neurons in the spinal cord of the elderly, and this is believed to be a factor that contributes to their muscle atrophy. According to Eugenia Wang of the University of Louisville, in Kentucky, an atrophying muscle provides a hostile environment for muscle repair and regeneration. Young muscle fibrils, or fiber parts, die when grafted onto an old, degenerating muscle. This is in contrast to the supportive environment that young, growing muscle provides for muscle repair. Fibrils from an old muscle will survive when grafted onto young muscle. Other factors needed to support the health of muscles are good blood flow and adequate nutrition, in the form of protein intake, to provide the amino acids used to build muscle. Good sources of protein are lean meat, whey and other dairy products, and nuts, especially almonds.

Exercise and Growth Hormone

Walking about in normal gravity has a major influence on the production and secretion of growth hormone. This hormone, which is so important in keeping up muscle mass, is reduced both in space and in bed-rest or prolonged inactivity. Growth hormone pours out after a bout of exercise. This does not happen either during spaceflight or during bed-rest of fourteen days duration, and the hormone is still absent for a few days after returning to Earth or to normal activity. But after four days of recovery, with the astronauts or bed-rest volunteers up and about once more, the growth hormone's response to exercise is restored.

What Can You Do about It?

Many of us would like somebody to invent a pill or a cream that will allow us to stay trim and firm without the need to exercise or maintain a good diet. All kinds of substances are touted, and sold, as miracle solutions. The results have been mixed at best. Health-food stores and suppliers selling through the internet readily offer anabolic substances and nutritional supplements with all-embracing claims that they will give you stronger muscles, make wrinkles disappear, lower your blood pressure and cholesterol, and increase your libido—all with no adverse side effects. There are no reliable studies to substantiate many of their claims, though the psychological benefit of believing something will help may be potent. In some cases, there are considerable benefits, but if taken to excess, some supplements could also have damaging effects. What they also do not tell you is that most do not work if you are not active.

What Works, What Doesn't?

Can the consequences of time or neglect be reversed? If astronauts recover after returning from space, so can you. Muscles of the back and even those of the neck and face can be firmed up—something no cream alone will ever do. But it is not going to happen without work and thought. Just as you have to read labels to know what you are eating, you also have to understand what and how different exercises, drugs, hormones, and supplements act so you can choose wisely. It is important to bear in mind that variety is the key to keeping you motivated. It is also the key to keeping your muscles from becoming bored and non-responsive. Remember to stretch and warm up before you start in order to avoid injuries. Stretching and warming up are important even if you do not exercise. If you stretch first thing in the morning, starting even before you get out of bed, you will protect your body from injury caused by such everyday activities as twisting, lifting heavy objects, or just getting out of bed. If you do exercise, you must allow your muscles time to recover between bouts, depending on the activity. This is why weight training is recommended only two or three times a week, whereas you can walk every day.

Remedies supposed to maintain or restore muscle health fall into three categories: physiological (substances that naturally occur in the body), pharmacological (drugs), and physical.

Physiological Remedies

These include a range of hormones, trace metals, and vitamins. Growth hormone and sex steroids build up muscle. But there are also risks. Other hormones break muscle down and some supplements seem to have no effect at all and are a waste of your money.

Growth Hormone

Growth hormone is advertised on the internet and elsewhere as a cure-all for the ills that come with aging. Most of the benefits they mention are indeed based on research results but usually in experimental animals, given large doses for short periods of time. There are many things you are not told. Large doses have been found to produce cardiovascular complications. It is always a good idea to check with your doctor before you take it.

One of the disadvantages of growth hormone is that it must be injected. It will not work if taken by mouth, because it is broken down in the stomach. Many ineffective or less effective variations of growth hormone are being sold and used without prescription. Their source and potency are unknown, and some could therefore have harmful side effects. If growth hormone must be used, it should be done so under the supervision of a physician. Trans-dermal patches are now being tested as a means of making it more convenient to take.

If you want to get the best benefits out of growth hormone, you need to exercise while you are taking it. NASA research has found that even very large doses of growth hormone given to experimental animals do not completely prevent muscle atrophy caused by inactivity. However, very small amounts of this hormone completely prevent muscle atrophy if combined with even light exercise. This is a highly significant discovery that is finding new applications in the world of medicine. AIDS patients, who suffer the complication of severe muscle wasting, are being helped to maintain muscle mass with light doses of growth hormone and light exercise.

Steroids

Anabolic steroids (such as sex steroids), which stimulate the building of protein, can increase the mass of atrophied muscles. Unfortunately, this property is also used to enhance athletic performance. Now even more potent synthetic relatives of these steroids, such as THG (tetrahydrogestrinone), designed to be undetectable in blood and urine, are being made available to athletes, with serious consequences to their health as well as to sport ethics.

The illegal use of androgenic steroids in the United States has been estimated at almost 1% in men and 0.1% in women, but among twelfth graders—seventeen to eighteen-year-olds—it was as high as 3.2% in 1996 and 4.5% in 2003. Its use is probably even more common than these figures indicate, because it can be bought at health-food stores. In sufficiently high amounts, the harmful effects are similar to those of testosterone in adults, but they may be far more serious in adolescents.

Catabolic steroids (such as cortisol), which break protein down, are the by-product of unmanaged stress or given as treatment in conditions of inflammation and allergic reaction. They have profound negative effects on muscle, as well as bone, joints, and skin. Even when applied locally they make skin papery thin.

• Sex Steroids: Testosterone

Testosterone is the hormone that fuels the male sex drive. It also plays a key role in building up muscle. Throughout human history, testes, extracts from them, and, when they were discovered, male sex steroids (androgens) have been the most popular source of rejuvenation cures in clinics and spas. Aging can be accompanied by a decline in the amount of testosterone in the blood, although many older men can have normal or near-normal testosterone levels. Disease-related problems, stress, malnutrition, and medications may also lower testosterone levels. In addition, the response of the testes to the pituitary hormones that regulate them is diminished in older men. Until fairly recently, reducing the influence of gravity and inactivity were generally not considered to affect testosterone. However, we now know that stays of several months in space result in reduced testosterone levels in healthy astronauts and cosmonauts.

Even if you have enough testosterone, inactivity will decrease the sensitivity of muscle to this hormone. Researchers at the Pennington Institute, in Louisiana, studied the effect of testosterone treatment on muscle mass and metabolism in healthy men in their twenties. The positive effects of testosterone in muscle building did not occur when these young men were made inactive by bed-rest for thirty days. The sensitivity of muscle to testosterone in older men has not been studied. However, testosterone replacement over a three-year period in men whose blood levels of the hormone were lower than normal was much more effective in increasing muscle strength in the young than it was for a group of elderly men.

There is no direct equivalent in men of the female menopause, because there is no acute drop in testosterone levels but only a gradual decline with age. However, testosterone skin patches are now being discussed for use in what is called the *andropause*. There seems to be no justification for taking testosterone unless it is to replace a significant decrease. Like any other hormone taken to excess, testosterone taken for bodybuilding can have toxic effects, as can other androgens that are converted to testosterone. Cardiovascular disease is the most serious of these. One theory holds that the increase in cardiovascular disease in women after the menopause is not necessarily due to the reduction of estrogen but may be the result of a relative increase in androgens. In older men, testosterone administration can stimulate an undesirable and dangerous growth of the prostate gland.

• Sex Steroids: DHEA

Dehydroepiandrosterone (DHEA) is a steroid hormone produced by the adrenal gland. It achieved notoriety in the 1960s as a supposed cure-all for stress. More recently, the alleviation of age-related illnesses, including diabetes, obesity, heart problems, and Alzheimer's disease, has been added to its list of benefits. However, it has also been correlated with an increased risk of breast cancer in women, a higher incidence of cardiovascular problems in men and women, and a suppressed immune response in the elderly.

In the body, it is normally converted into the sex steroids, testosterone in males and estrogen in females. DHEA levels increase progressively, starting at five to seven years of age and reaching a peak in the twenties, after which they gradually decline then go into a steeper decline after age eighty. Claims of the benefits brought about by DHEA remain unsubstantiated.

• Sex Steroids: Androstenedione

Androstenedione is formed from DHEA before being converted to estrogen or testosterone. Like DHEA, androstenedione has also been marketed primarily to athletes and to bodybuilders. Because very high doses of testosterone have been shown to increase muscle mass and strength, it was assumed that androstenedione would have similar anabolic effects. However, although the level of testosterone does increase after androstenedione is taken, the size of the increase is too small for protein synthesis, and therefore muscle mass, to increase. Controlled studies have been limited, but in general they do not point to any beneficial effects.

• Catabolic Steroids: Learn How to Manage Stress

The best way to conserve muscle is to avoid things that break it down. Next to inactivity, stress must be avoided. Just as activity improves the positive muscle-building effects of growth hormone and testosterone, so does inactivity heighten the negative effects of catabolic hormones, such as cortisol. This hormone is put out naturally during times of stress or trauma, and its effect is even more harmful if the person is bedridden. Healthy volunteers in bed for fourteen days suffered three times as much muscle loss after taking a single dose of cortisol as when they were up and about.

Though cortisol can be a lifesaver when prescribed for allergic conditions and inflammation of the joints, it does break down both muscle and bone and should only be used for short periods. Learning how to manage stress is the best way of keeping one's cortisol levels in check.

Vitamins and Other Supplements
• Creatine

This is a popular nutritional supplement on shop shelves that promises to deliver improved lean body mass and better results from exercise. The powder, mixed with food and taken orally, is supposed to work by increasing the amount of chemical energy available for muscle contraction. However, studies comparing creatine with a placebo, with or without exercise training, failed to confirm these claims.

• Chromium Picolinate

Supplements of the trace element chromium, in the form of chromium picolinate, have also been claimed to increase lean body mass, muscle size, and strength. A clinical test in older men who participated in resistance training for twelve weeks found no added benefit of this substance.

Physical Interventions

Physical interventions include the electrical stimulation of muscles, exercise, and increased gravity loading.

• Electrical Stimulation

Nerve connections are critical to the health of muscle and bone because they carry electrical and chemical messages. But the amount of electrical activity reaching muscle is reduced with inactivity or with aging. Electrical stimulation of muscle (EMS) is therefore considered as a treatment for wasting muscles. In polio victims and some spinal-cord injury patients, it is used to maintain muscle function and mass.

Soviet scientists successfully tested EMS as a treatment in preventing muscle atrophy in cosmonauts during spaceflight. In our research, daily EMS of the leg muscles of healthy volunteers in bed-rest for thirty days also proved useful in preventing atrophy and loss of muscle tone. The level of electrical stimulation different individuals can tolerate varies considerably. EMS forces muscles to contract when they can no longer do so naturally. Less current is needed to stimulate a nerve to create a muscle contraction than to stimulate the muscle directly. EMS methods have varied considerably. As many as ten to twenty electrodes are used at different points on a leg muscle, the amount of current ranging from 1–30 mA (milliamp) intensity. The duration of treatment may last from fifteen minutes to several hours a day. Currents that persist for about one second are most often used.

Exercise

Lack of time, money, and easy access to fitness facilities are frequent reasons for not exercising. These obstacles can be overcome, so long as there is no lack of motivation.

Many are put off by the popular misconception that many hours of intense exercise are required for significant gain. The President's Council on Physical Fitness recommends a "no pain, no gain" approach. However, it can be even more effective to exercise by using a variety of slow moves of high intensity, properly designed and supervised and correctly performed, as long as this is part of a daily routine of activity that uses gravity to its fullest.

Any exercise is better than none. Each day, it is essential to give some work to just about every muscle in the body. Those that specifically use gravity involve using the body's weight or carrying additional weights. However, not all exercise is equally effective. Doing the exercise correctly, using the right form and speed, can make the difference between tremendous benefit or very little. Each exercise targets a specific muscle or muscle group. There seems to be no better way than physical activity to keep muscles healthy throughout life.

Exercising means you are contracting your muscles. Muscles get stronger when you make them work: walking, gardening, going up or down stairs, dancing, or house cleaning all help. If you have not gardened for a while, even if you walk or bicycle daily, your unused muscles soon let you know it once you pick up a garden fork and set to work. The benefits of sudden enthusiastic bursts of exercise are lost very much faster than they are gained. It is also simplistic to believe you can reverse muscle loss and maintain fitness by pottering around the garden once in a while or doing exercises in a chair where the effect of gravity is reduced.

There are two basic types of exercise, aerobic and anaerobic. Aerobic exercise relies on increasing the amount of oxygen taken in. JoAnn Manson and her group at the Harvard School of Public Health, in Boston, found women who walked briskly at least three hours per week or did other vigorous exercise for one and a half hours per week were 30 to 40% less likely to get coronary heart disease. Along the same lines, a study of 21,000 male physicians who exercised enough to a sweat once per week found a 24% reduction in the risk of Type-2 diabetes. Exercising two to four times per week reduced their risk by 39%. The key word here is "sweat." Aerobic exercise is most useful in keeping the cardiovascular system fit and in stimulating the metabolic rate.

Anaerobic exercise, on the other hand, uses energy stored in the muscles in the form of carbohydrates. It includes repeating activities of such intensity that you can only maintain them for short periods—less than two minutes. No exercise or sport involves purely one or the other. In general, however, explosive events, such as sprinting and weightlifting, are anaerobic and endurance events, such as long-distance running, are aerobic. Football, tennis, walking, cycling, and baseball can be both, because they can involve sustained effort or combine short periods of intense activity with periods of recovery. As you get older you can reach the same level of intensity that you did in your younger days, but it takes longer to recover. So make sure you allow yourself time for that recovery.

How long should you exercise for? The consensus among exercise physiologists now is that small bursts of aerobic exercise, weight training, or flexibility training—eight or ten minutes, repeated several times throughout the day—will bring the same benefits as setting aside half an hour a day for a solid block of exercise. This is important, because the excuse people who do not exercise most often give is that they cannot find the time. It is usually easier to fit in a few eight-minute sessions than to set aside half an hour.

• Stretching and Flexibility

Before you even start any exercise, even housework, you need to warm up and stretch your muscles. Have you watched Olympic sprinters warming up for the 100-meter dash? Although they are at peak fitness, they will stretch and warm up their muscles for a long time before an effort that will last for just ten seconds or less. Flexibility diminishes significantly with age, though not all parts of the body lose flexibility at the same rate. Connective tissue becomes less elastic. Stretching acts as a stimulus to connective tissue. Stretching exercises have been shown to increase the flexibility and range of motion of knee joints, ankles, and the lower back and to reduce aches and pains in those joints.

If you are off your feet for a good part of the day you will find, as the astronauts did, that the soles of your feet are tender when you first step on them in the morning. Before you even get out of bed, stretch the way you used to as a child. Stretch your arms over your head while pulling your legs and feet in the opposite direction at the same time. Make yourself as tall as possible. Give your ankles a good workout: turn your feet in and out, then up and down, and rotate them a dozen times in each direction. You will find taking that first step does not hurt quite as much.

Unlike other exercises, stretching does not promote fat loss. However, it is very helpful in preventing injury, especially if done before and after other more intensive activities.

• Strength Training

When the muscles that support the body have lost their strength or begin to fade away, the most effective way of reviving them is to keep them in a state of heightened tension. Charles Atlas fans knew this as "dynamic tension." Contracting a muscle and holding the contraction, lifting weights and holding them, or pushing against resistance for several minutes will keep muscles in this state of heightened tension. The body's muscles that counteract gravity do that automatically when you are standing to maintain your posture against gravity.

Weight training cannot be done in space, where neither the body nor any other physical object has any weight. However, resistance exercise can be partially effective there in maintaining both muscle mass and strength. On Earth, gravity provides a great advantage. It is always there, so you can do weight training at any moment during the day. Weight training has now been shown to have the added benefit of increasing aerobic capacity as well.

Descriptions of resistance exercises, also called strength training, can be found in an excellent guide that can be obtained free from the National Institute on Aging in Maryland. *Exercise: A Guide from the National Institute on Aging and the National Aeronautics and Space Administration* was published in 1998 on the occasion of John Glenn's second trip to space. The high and sustained isometric tension developed within the muscle increases blood pressure without increasing blood flow. For this reason, strength training was until recently not recommended for the elderly, who often have high blood pressure, and there was concern that resistance exercise could be dangerous. A number of studies have now examined the benefits of such exercise and found no adverse consequences.

• Good Posture

Not making the effort to maintain good posture can make even a young person look stooped and old. Slouching is essentially giving in to gravity, allowing it to pull us down. In Victorian times, corsets, profuse skirts, flounced underskirts, and straight-backed chairs necessitated good posture. But modern dress and habits make for sloppy posture. Mitchell A. Mabardy, a World War II veteran with many injuries and surgical repairs, came to exercise at ninety-four at my fitness club in Alexandria, Virginia. After completing his routine on the machines, he showered. Then he returned to the aerobics room, where, dressed in his blue blazer and surrounded by mirrors, he methodically walked around, checking that he was holding himself upright. In fact, have you ever noticed that the dynamic elderly in the over-eighty age group, even some centenarians, are those with the best posture? They sit, stand, walk, and hold themselves tall in a way that many younger people have yet to learn.

The head accounts for 17% of the body's entire weight. Neck pain, upper back pain, and serious orthopedic problems result if it is not properly supported because the muscles designed to support it are not kept fit.

Low back pain, hip problems, and knee problems result from under-exercised abdominal and lower back muscles; the body's weight is allowed to sink as it is pulled down by gravity and the weight of a sagging abdomen. Most of today's armchairs and sofas are designed in a way that encourages slouching. The neck muscles cannot support the head, because it is no longer positioned straight above the torso, so the slouching becomes progressively worse and the spine starts curving. The remedy is to remember to stand and sit tall and hold your stomach in—and to change your chair!

• Pilates Exercises

Strong abdominal muscles are crucial for a healthy back. Strengthening exercises for the relatively small back muscles that support the spine are useful but not nearly as critical as toning of the large lower abdominal muscles. One of this group that is commonly neglected, because it is not easy to exercise, is the transverse abdominus, a big muscle that runs across the base of the abdomen and wraps all the way around to your back. It keeps your intestines and other organs in place. When it sags it pulls your spine forward or sideways, a major cause of back pain and slipped discs. This is the muscle that contracts when you give a hearty belly laugh, exhale hard, or sneeze.

The best exercise to tone the muscles of the trunk of your body is core-training, also known as Pilates exercises. Joseph Pilates (1880–1967), a German citizen interned in England in World War I, pioneered a technique that allowed wounded soldiers lying in bed to exercise their trunk muscles and keep themselves in good shape. This conditioning regimen also served to improve posture and muscle strength, enabling the soldiers to get back to the battlefield sooner. It also has a long history of use by dancers and has been rediscovered by the fitness gurus in the last five years. Several disciples of Pilates, now in their eighties, continue to practice and to train others. The concept has once again become very popular. To find authorized Pilates instructors in your area, look up the official website, www.pilates-studio.com.

The exercises—leg and spine stretches, modified sit-ups, push-ups, and leg and arm exercises while exhaling forcefully and deeply at the same time—are all designed to engage the transverse abdominus. Instead of many quick repetitions, movements are slow, with few repetitions. The benefits depend on learning to keep the abdominal muscles contracted at all times to strengthen them and help you maintain good posture.

Exercises that work the abdominal and lower back muscles and those that support the shoulder blades, neck, and upper spine are best at improving posture. Keep your stomach muscles contracted whenever you think of it and you will go a long way toward making it a good habit. I try to do these exercises when waiting at traffic lights, watching television, or sitting in front of a computer. Couple these contractions with a forced exhalation, emptying your lungs as much as possible, and you will be working your elusive lower abdominal muscles as well.

• Toning Up Your Face and Neck Muscles: Whistle Power

The muscles of the face and those under the chin are among the most visible casualties of gravity. The lower jaw muscles are very much affected by gravity. Making an effort to pronounce things clearly and to chew food thoroughly and deliberately will help those facial muscles. Unpleasant as it is to watch, chewing gum is not a bad facial muscle-toning exercise. Professional opera singers take voice and elocution lessons and rarely show sagging cheeks.

Whistling is one of the most effective ways to tone up the facial muscles. What a shame that we seem to quit whistling as we get older. Whistling is enjoyable, requires no expensive equipment, and does wonders for good breathing as well.

A good exercise for the front neck muscles can be done lying in bed on your back with your head hanging slightly over but still supported by the bed. Raise your head slowly, until it is level with your body. This is a very small movement, but you should feel it in the front of the neck. Hold it there for a slow count of three, breathing naturally. Relax your head back. Repeat six times. As your neck muscles get stronger, you can try hanging your head further out, off the end of the bed, to increase your range of motion, but always bring your head slowly in line with your body. Never jerk your head. This works neck muscles against the force of gravity, using the weight of the head to strengthen the muscles.

If all else fails you can hide those crinkled neck skin wrinkles with good posture—shoulders down, long neck, head up, chin down.

• Hypergravity

If doing individual exercises with separate weights for each muscle you want to target takes too much time and effort, you may soon be able to try "whole-body weight training." I call it that because by doubling your body weight, every movement you make involves twice as much work. The theory behind it is that a ride on a centrifuge increases the gravity load and hence the body's weight. Muscles and bones that support body weight and respond to loading would be expected to benefit most from such a challenge. As yet, only the prototype of a machine I developed for this purpose is available, at NASA's Ames Research Center, in California. It is being evaluated for its use in keeping astronauts healthy on the way to Mars. But you may one day be able to cut the time it takes to do your daily workout by enjoying a centrifuge ride while going through your favorite resistance exercise routine at twice Earth's gravity, and hence twice your body weight.

Reversing Aging: The Fitness Revolution

The myth that muscle wastes away irreversibly with age is broken. Geriatrician Maria Fiatarone Singh and her colleagues at the Tufts University, Hebrew Rehabilitation Center, in Boston, Massachusetts, showed in a 1994 cornerstone study that muscle weakness in the elderly was reversible. Increases in muscle strength and endurance were achieved after twelve weeks' training with weights, in men and women as old as ninety. They could safely lift weights that were previously thought to be beyond them. A doubling in strength was reported for some of the muscle groups trained in this manner. Lifting weights also restored bone density. Even more impressive were their increased energy levels, renewed ability to walk and take care of themselves, and general sense of emotional well-being. Several studies have now confirmed these findings. If they can do it, anyone can.

Until this study was done, muscle wasting and bone loss were considered the inevitable and irreversible consequences of aging. Not surprisingly, it started an unprecedented interest in exercise among the elderly, once thought to be too frail to participate. Senior fitness classes graduated from stretching to pumping iron. It is no longer unusual to see a senior at a Nautilus leg-press machine at the local YMCA. Nursing homes and community centers are introducing weight-training classes at a rapid rate.

Wayne Westcott, fitness director at the South Shore YMCA in Quincy, Massachusetts, developed a program based on a 1996 study of 1,132 people aged twenty to eighty. Not only did the sixty to eighty-year-olds gain muscle and maintain it with consistent workouts, but in terms of improvement they did as well as the forty to sixty and even the twenty to forty-year-olds. He estimates more than a hundred nursing homes nationwide now offer such strength-building programs. Beverly Enterprises of Fort Smith, Arkansas, have been introducing this program throughout their 550 long-term care facilities, which they operate nationwide.

There is a veritable revolution going on in the fitness world, with seniors demanding and winning attention as never before. The American Senior Fitness Association accredits trainers specializing in exercise for seniors. Nautilus, Keiser Corporation, and other equipment providers are designing devices that add weight in 1-lb increments rather than the usual 5-lb steps found in most fitness clubs. Manufacturers and retailers are courting the senior market with attractive, comfortable sportswear. The *1996 Surgeon General's Report on Physical Activity and Health* recommends muscle-strengthening exercise as part of an overall exercise-training regime for older adults. Gravity is what makes these exercises effective. Seniors are on the march!

Keeping the Engine Tuned

The brain is the control center of the body. Through its branches—the spinal cord and the network of nerves—it communicates, receives signals and information from outside the body, and then evaluates, organizes, and directs the appropriate response. Too loud a noise, we cover our ears. Too hot, we sweat. If we lift an arm against the pull of gravity, muscles contract to make it possible. When the brain senses increased blood volume, it orchestrates a response to reduce it.

The nervous system must remain tuned and responsive to function at its best. To do that it requires stimulation—that is, a series of challenges, with time allowed between them for recovery. The frequency, intensity, and the pattern of the stimulus determine how effective it will be. Body systems have evolved to use gravity as that stimulus.

To keep the body's systems tuned and the senses sharp, it is important that the challenges be intermittent. For if the stimulus is constant, the body simply adapts to it. Step into a chocolate shop and you will immediately be aware of the lovely aroma, but work in one and soon you will no longer smell it.

The importance of this stimulation is to keep all systems working within a small range of limits, like a thermostat that kicks in when the temperature drops below the setting and turns off when it exceeds it. Such tuning keeps blood-pressure sensors sensitive and memory and reaction time sharp. Hormone and immune systems must be responsive and balance and coordination of movements primed, ready to prevent a fall.

Fine tuning is needed to synchronize the body's clock and its relationship to its environment. The proper regulation of body rhythms, or ensuring a refreshing night's sleep, depends primarily on light and gravity, but also on meals, activity, sexual activity, social interaction, and combinations of these.

A well-tuned nervous system determines the body's ability to respond.

4

The Senses, Balance, and Coordination

His head must know where his head is.

—*Gustav Eckstein, (1890-1981), The Body Has a Head*

In the early days of the space program, Soviet cosmonauts reported feeling sick almost as soon as they got into space, whereas "our boys," the U.S. astronauts, did not. It was thought that perhaps the smaller Mercury and Gemini capsules, where they had no room to move about, protected them from this unpleasant experience. The story goes that during the *Gemini 7* mission in 1965, the intercom was accidentally left on and Jim Lovell was heard to chide Frank Borman about making sure he used the barf bag. The secret was out!

Later in the program, with a greater amount of room to move about in the Apollo capsule, on Skylab, on the Shuttle, and now on the Space Station, 50–75% of the U.S. crews report experiencing space sickness. This ranges from what they describe as "stomach awareness" to vomiting that lasts the first two to three days. This is the perfect example of what may be the result of a conflict in the information the senses receive. The eyes see a floor and a ceiling in the spacecraft, but in the near-zero gravity of space the body does not sense an up or down.

On returning to Earth, there is a new set of conflicting conditions. Astronauts again feel disoriented and sometimes nauseous. However, they adapt once more and recover within a few days. But it takes longer for them to regain their sense of balance and walk again, which they did not need to do in space.

Sudden changes in sensory input, like that of first going into space, are not encountered often on Earth and are therefore not a problem as we get older. However, just as it is with astronauts, unsteady balance and poor coordination of

71

movements are certainly two of the earliest and most important symptoms that have come to be associated with getting older. The consequences of taking a fall and breaking a thinning bone could be catastrophic.

Without gravity, the brain and the systems it controls show many more signs of deterioration normally associated with aging. These range from slower response of muscles to nerve impulses, a falling off in the ability of the heart and blood vessels to cope with the demands made on them, disturbed sleep, poor appetite, or a decreased sense of thirst. Other problems we associate with aging, such as loss of hearing, failing eyesight, memory lapses, reduced attention span, inability to cope with stress, and feelings of aloneness and depression, are likely to be seen in longer flights, such as trips to Mars. However, astronauts will soon recover when back on Earth.

In May 1998, NASA launched *Neurolab STS-90*, a sixteen-day Shuttle mission, as its contribution to the Decade of the Brain. It was dedicated to research on the brain and nervous system. Together with the mission of *STS-95*, when John Glenn returned to space on the Shuttle in October 1998, these flights were a valuable beginning in uncovering the role of gravity on brain function as we develop and age.

How the System Works

Lift an arm, lie down, open your mouth to say a few words and you activate a network of around 100 billion nerve cells in the brain. Not much bigger than a cauliflower, the brain is the most complex structure in the human body. It is the prompter of action, the seat of consciousness, intelligence, memory, imagination, and the emotions, as well as the site where pleasure, pain, vision, taste, hearing, and other sensations are registered.

Along with the spinal cord, the brain is the control center for the rest of the body. Brain cells, or neurons, receive electrical and chemical messages, through thread-like extensions called dendrites, and decide whether or not to pass them on, through extensions known as axons. Between an axon and a dendrite there is a gap called a synapse, and the signal gets across this gap by means of a chemical known as a transmitter.

Protected by the bony shell of the skull and cushioned by three membranes with fluid between them, the brain receives and analyzes messages from the sense organs. It checks them against its database of experience, decides what to do about them, and passes "action this moment" commands to thousands of other cells in the body. Messages flash from neuron to neuron and to their final destinations in the split second it takes to blink an eye. The brain's central importance can be gauged from the fact that in the average adult it accounts for about 2% of bodyweight yet demands 20% of the body's blood supply.

Five Senses—or More?

The senses are the brain's link with the environment—the reality that surrounds us. Traditionally we recognize five: touch, taste, smell, hearing, and vision. Sensory organs such as the eyes, ears, nose, skin, and taste buds are specialized to receive stimuli from the physical world and transmit them to the brain by nerve impulses. We also have what has been described as a "sixth sense," located in the inner ear and in what are known as proprioceptors, in muscles, skin, tendons, and joints. They can even be found in the soles of the feet. They receive stimuli from gravity and from acceleration and transmit them to the brain. Pilots who talk about "flying by the seat of their pants" are referring to these proprioceptors. There may even be a "seventh sense." Scientists have discovered a photopigment in the retina of the eye, called melanopsin, that is not involved with vision but receives light signals that are important in synchronizing the body's daily rhythms.

The Miraculous Mechanism of the Inner Ear

The system that controls our ability to stand and move is one of the most elegant and complicated in the body. Understanding how it works helps us recognize what we can do to keep it in top condition. The brain evolved to use the downward-pulling force of gravity in a body that can orient itself by moving in different directions. The first requirement is an apparatus that will sense the direction and characteristics of the gravity stimulus. This is found in the inner ear, protected by the skull and close to the part of the ear concerned with hearing. The structures of the ear are organized into three distinct regions: the outer ear, middle ear, and inner ear. The first region extends from outside the body to the eardrum, which vibrates when it is hit by sound waves. The middle ear is an air-filled chamber containing three tiny bones that transmit and amplify sound from the eardrum. The sense of hearing is located in the inner ear, where the waving motion of thousands of tiny hair cells in the spiraling, snail-like cochlea sends nerve signals to the brain. The inner ear also contains the vestibular system, which controls our sense of balance.

The Ear's Vestibular System

The purpose of the vestibular system is to receive and transmit to the brain information about the position and motion of the head relative to gravity and also about the head's direction and speed of movement. It is called "vestibular" because it consists of several chambers, or vestibules, strategically positioned at various angles to each other. All share a common type of cell, a hair cell that receives and transmits information to the brain.

The Inner Ear

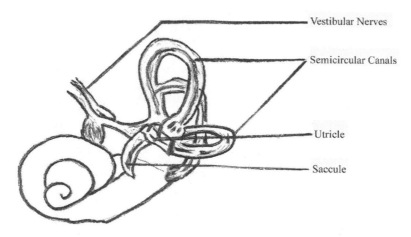

Vestibular Nerves

Semicircular Canals

Utricle

Saccule

This diagram shows the vestibular system of the inner ear.

Within the vestibular system are three fluid-filled semicircular canals, or membranous tubes, embedded in a bony structure of the same shape. They are positioned roughly at right angles to each other and their job is to pick up any rotation of the head, whether up and down, tilting side to side towards the shoulders or turning sideways, or left and right. As you move your head, fluid moves inside the tube that lies in the plane of the movement. As it swishes, it causes the hairs on the hair cells to bend ever so slightly. This movement stimulates the hair cell to send messages to the brain, reporting the bending. If you rotate your head, spinning in the form of motion known as angular acceleration, and suddenly stop, the fluid swishes back in the opposite direction. This causes dizziness. In space, angular acceleration continues in the absence of gravity and is felt every time an astronaut tumbles or turns. The semicircular canals of astronauts, then, are not affected in space.

The vestibular system also contains two more chambers, the utricle and the saccule, collectively called the *otolith organs*. Otolith means "ear stone" in Greek. They are called that because instead of fluid, the hairs are covered by a gel within which are embedded tiny grains of calcium carbonate crystals, similar to grains of sand. If the head moves in one plane forward and back or up and down, as in a jump, the grains in the gel move across the hair cells, bending the hairs, which in turn alert the cell to send signals to the brain. The otolith organs pick up these linear head movements. Because of its place in the vestibular system, the saccule is more sensitive to vertical acceleration, such as going up and down in an elevator or diving and jumping, while the utricle picks up the kind of horizontal acceleration we experience when riding in a car. Riding a roller coaster stimulates both.

In practical terms, we think of space as being a region of zero gravity. In fact, gravity still operates in space, though its strength is vastly reduced. Even though their spacecraft is moving, astronauts in space are unaware of linear acceleration, because it registers only movements against the force of gravity. The otoliths detect some linear acceleration every time an astronaut pushes off the side of the spacecraft wall and perceives the contact force when an astronaut, secured by bungee cords, exercises on a treadmill. However, that's all. The stimulus is extremely weak, and as a result the otoliths become less sensitive. This is not a problem until the astronauts return to Earth.

How the System Perceives Signals

Signals from vestibular hair cells are transmitted to the brain through nerve fibers and result in an internal representation of the position of the head during movement. The brain is the human central-processing unit. It operates all the time, day and night. The brain uses this information, along with messages from the eyes, ears, and the sense of touch, to tell the muscles what to do in order to maintain balance. Watch an ice skater land elegantly after a triple lutz and you are watching the senses concerned with balance in operation at their most awesome and spectacular pitch.

The senses that work in concert with the vestibular system become particularly important if the vestibular system itself is damaged or impaired. This can happen through infection of the ear, as a result of drugs, or because the system has been unused in the reduced gravity of space or because of an over-sedentary lifestyle. If you ask an astronaut just returned from space, or an older person, to stand on a swaying platform with their eyes open, they will do well enough. Ask them to close their eyes and they quickly lose their balance.

Just as the eyes complement the vestibular system, so does the vestibular system help to stabilize the eyes. The vestibulo-ocular reflex, as it is called, enables us to move our heads up and down or sideways while our gaze remains fixed on an object straight ahead. A newborn child tilted backwards rolls its eyes downward so that its gaze remains fixed. This is a natural reflex in the presence of gravity. The body compensates for the change in orientation and the response is partly controlled by the vestibular system in the inner ear.

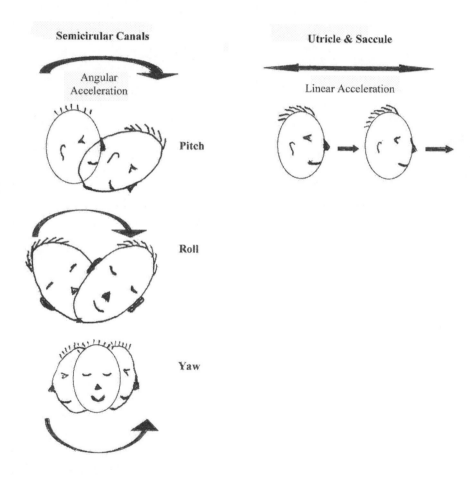

This diagram indicates the type of motion that stimulates semicircular canals, or the utricle and saccule. Pitching the head forward (pitch), rolling it from side to side (roll), or rotating it to either side (yaw) induces angular acceleration that stimulates the semicircular canals. Linear acceleration, by moving forward, stimulates the utricle and saccule.

Where in the World Are We?

In addition to the balancing mechanism of the inner ear, and to the senses of vision and hearing, our ability to sense our position in relation to our surroundings depends on the proprioceptors, a network of motion, pressure, and temperature sensors in the muscles, joints, tendons, and skin. Proprioceptors provide the brain's processing unit with information about the sensation of the loading of the limbs as they bear the weight of the body and of the movement, stretching, or contraction and position of muscles, joints, and limbs. Any condition that affects weight distribution, muscle mass, tendon status, or the junction of nerve and muscle will also alter reflexes and our awareness of the position of body, head, and limbs.

The integration of all this incoming information by the brain is in effect translated into an internal diagram of the position of all parts of the body in relation to surrounding space. This internal brain map, rather like the moving three-dimensional models that give information to an air-traffic controller, comes in the form of a *pattern of place*, neurons firing in certain locations in the hippocampus corresponding exactly with our three-dimensional space. The hippocampus is a small structure at the base of the brain that plays a major role in memory and in the integration of information. The resultant "brain map" gives us precise control over movements of the eyes, head, arms, legs, and body.

What Can Go Wrong?

Balance and Coordination

It is believed that 65% of elderly people in the U.S. die as a result of an injury related to a fall. Not only does the likelihood of a fall become greater with age, but its consequences can be far more serious. Why is this so? The inability to stand firmly could be due to muscle atrophy, to changes in the sharpness of our reflexes, and to a loss or diminution of the sense of balance. In general, people who realize they have some difficulty standing or walking automatically compensate by altering their stance and holding their feet wider apart to keep their center of gravity closer to the ground. Yet again, it is not the passing of the years that affects the sense of balance; it is using the gravity stimulus to keep the system tuned.

Watching the seventy-seven-year-old John Glenn come down the Shuttle steps after *STS 95* landed on July 18, 1998, reminded me of babies learning to stand up and walk. He stood with his feet wide apart and walked tentatively.

Many astronauts in both the U.S. and the Russian programs have been unsteady on their legs for the first few days after returning to Earth. They walk with their feet wide apart and take short strides. Their ability to land properly when asked to jump is also impaired. They show a tendency to fall to the outside when turning corners, sometimes bumping into the walls. They also lose their ability to pick up each foot properly and place it down heel first.

The process of programming the brain in a baby so that it learns how to stand, walk, and run is very similar to that of reprogramming an astronaut's brain on returning to Earth's gravity from space. First the brain must sense and recognize the direction of gravity, and then it must send commands to the body to make the most efficient movements with respect to gravity in order to stay upright and move about. Although the brains of astronauts, like those of the earthbound majority, are programmed to do this from childhood, they have not had to use this balance and coordination system while in space. Suddenly back in gravity, they behave as if the memory of what to do has been lost and their brains have to relearn or recall the process.

The same can be true in the elderly, who may not have kept up activities that keep the balance and coordination systems in prime condition. As we begin to realize that our ability to control movement is declining, we tend to venture out less, and when we do we are much more apprehensive. Eventually, this spiral of compromised activity affects our quality of life and results in disability. There is often a lower desire for purposeful activity or even a reluctance to leave the house. Observations from our bed-rest studies reinforce this belief. Young, healthy men after sixteen or thirty days in head-down bed-rest step off the bed very tentatively, and just like the astronauts they stand and walk with their feet wide apart, take shorter strides, and have trouble negotiating corners. They also tend to shuffle, partly because after being off their feet for so many days their soles are tender and partly because they may have a problem placing their feet down in a normal manner.

Rats that return from fourteen days in space tend to drop and drag their feet when they first walk on the ground again. If you watch a baby learning to walk, it also first drags its feet before putting weight on them and stepping forward. Learning to walk requires that we first be exposed to the directional stimulus of gravity then have the equipment to sense it and finally the tools to respond to it.

A brain damaged at birth may require hypergravity, a higher intensity of gravity stimulus, before a child's brain becomes programmed to respond to direction and acceleration, senses necessary for walking. This would mean that rehabilitation exercises in children with cerebral palsy should be more effective if done in the upright position in a way that the body may experience some load, even if the child has to be supported by a harness. Alternately, the movement therapy could be done on a centrifuge.

The Compensating Brain

The brain has wonderful ways of developing strategies to make up for what may be missing. Jordan Grafman at the National Institute of Neurological Diseases and Stroke (NINDS), in Maryland, gives the example of compensatory strategies we use driving home or to work. One person may rely mainly on street signs, others on a general sense of direction and location without reading the signs, and some on a mixture of both. If a brain injury damages the ability to read signs, Grafman believes, the brain may shift to the more general approach of spatial location and a sense of direction. The brain compensates for any deficit by taking a different route or by growing new connections that bypass areas of damage, as in cases of stroke.

But this compensation, and the shift to a different strategy, may mask the damage and sometimes cause the injury to be underestimated. Inessa Kozlovskaya, one of my Russian colleagues, told me the story of a cosmonaut who had passed with flying colors the grueling battery of tests for space motion sickness, balance, and coordination. He flew on the Russian space station *Mir* for three months and was going through their rehabilitation program with his other two crewmates. After two months, his crewmates were well on the road to recovery, yet he was showing no progress. The medical team was perplexed and ran him through a set of tests that included Magnetic Resonance Imaging (MRI). The MRI showed he had a tumor on his cerebellum, the area of the brain that receives and integrates information and coordinates movements in response to gravity. Tumors in that region grow very slowly, so his brain had plenty of time to develop ways of compensating and bypassed the damaged area. But in space, he did not need to use these compensatory strategies, so on return to Earth he was left without the skills he had acquired. Away from the stimulus of gravity, his brain's memory of these strategies was erased. He unfortunately died during surgery to remove the tumor. Had he survived, the surgery, could he have recovered his balance and coordination? Chances were good that, given skilled and patient training, he would have learned or relearned compensatory strategies.

Changes in the control of movement in the elderly are very similar in kind to those seen in astronauts. They have usually been considered part and parcel of aging. But perhaps they are not. Owen Black, at the University of Oregon, observed that whereas there is a steady deterioration in balance and coordination until age eighty, there are measurable improvements in the over-eighty groups. Surely, balance and motor coordination do not suddenly improve after eighty. What the data strongly suggest is that those who maintain a lifestyle that keeps other diseases at bay will also maintain better balance and coordination of their movements and live longer. He found that he could relate progressive balance deterioration to the cumulative effect of bouts of disease.

Ever Get That Dizzy Feeling?

According to an analysis by the National Institute on Deafness and other Communication Disorders (NIDCD), in Maryland, about 6.2 million Americans experience balance problems or dizziness. About half of them are over sixty. However, the symptom of dizziness is not only due to inner-ear problems. Its causes can vary from low blood pressure, vision problems, stroke or head trauma to tumor, allergies, the effects of medication, and poor nutrition. Vertigo, the feeling that things around you are moving when they are not, can be brought about by the loosening of the calcium crystals in the inner ear and by degeneration of the vestibular system with age. It has therefore been suggested that it could be treated by rotating the person's head in such a way that the calcium crystals in the inner ear float back into place. This treatment is both difficult and controversial, and its effectiveness is impossible to prove.

As we get older, the subtle links between the vestibular system of the inner ear and the sense of vision (the vestibulo-ocular reflexes) also weaken. This affects our ability to maintain a steady gaze when we are moving. We first become aware of this when going up and down stairs. We may have to look at our feet when we walk, or we may get dizzy when we reach for something. Balance problems are not simple to diagnose and treat, so it is important to report any problem to a physician as soon as you become aware of it.

Peril on the Roads

With advancing age, driving becomes more challenging. The death rate among car drivers older than sixty-five is above average, and their accidents occur especially at intersections or when changing lanes. America's National Highway Safety Administration reported motorcycle deaths had jumped by more than a third between 1998 and 2000. This was at first attributed to ever-increasing engine sizes, allowing bikes to be driven ever faster. Most of the increase in deaths involved riders aged forty and over on bikes with engines larger than 1,000 cc. In 1990, the biggest motorbikes generally available had engines of 769 cc. With increasing engine size and plusher models, older riders tended to ride machines as powerful as they could afford. Unlike younger riders, they were less likely to die because of speeding, but most accidents involved balance problems when going round curves and changing lanes.

Balance Problems in Space and on Earth

In spaceflight, where there is neither up nor down, the brain receives far less information from the inner ear and the proprioceptors, the cells and nerve endings in the muscles, tendons, and joints that normally tell the body where it is in relation to the outside world. Sight and touch may tell the body that it is tilted, but the message from the inner ear is that there is no change. No wonder the brain is confused. It takes a few days for an astronaut to develop a new pattern of orientation, to use sensory information, and learn how to move around in space. Until this happens, signals are not interpreted properly, and the space traveler may feel disoriented and nauseous, sometimes to the point of vomiting. Space sickness during the first three or four days in flight is caused by this mismatch of signals, described as sensory conflict.

Although astronauts may see a floor and ceiling they have no inner sense of what either is. If they could not see their arms and legs, they would not know where these limbs were, because they have no weight to pass signals on to the brain. Astronauts working outside the spacecraft building the Space Station have nothing in their field of vision below them except for Earth hundreds of miles away. This leaves them in a potentially perilous situation, and some have reported a sense of falling even though they knew this was not happening.

We still have no good way of predicting who may or may not get sick in space, even after eliminating those candidates most liable to motion sickness by putting them through a formidable battery of tests. Individuals who do not get sick in any tests on the ground may become space sick, and vice versa. Just as with sea sickness, there is an element of conditioning, since rookie astronauts are more likely to get sick than experienced ones. Drugs used for motion sickness have had limited success.

Just as astronauts can be affected by vestibular dysfunction in space, so can ordinary earthbound people encounter balance problems as they grow older. But this is not inevitable, and it does not affect everybody. There is much that can be learned from spaceflight about sensing and processing gravity signals. Once the stimulus of gravity is removed, it becomes easier to understand how other stimuli operate. The brain is very adaptable, and in space it soon learns how to make do without gravity telling it which way is up. It is on returning to Earth that the problems begin.

A reduction in the ability to maintain a stable gaze, which may affect both astronauts in spaceflight and elderly people with vestibular disorders on Earth, can be measured by a visual-acuity test taken while walking on a treadmill. In both cases, those affected have blurred and unsteady vision. Techniques developed to test astronauts after returning from space also include using a platform that can gently sway forward and backward. Standing on such a platform, returning astronauts show greater sway and instability than they did before flight. If they close their eyes, they usually fall over, because their otolith system has lost its ability to take corrective action. I remember watching in amazement Rick Searfoss, who, after emerging from the *SLS-2* in December 1993, was standing on the sway platform being tested for balance. With eyes shut, he fell forward without even putting his arms out. He would have fallen flat on his face were it not for the support harness he was wearing.

Healthy volunteers who spend thirty days in head-down bed-rest also show increased sway on this "seesaw" platform. When they get out of bed they stand with their feet wide apart, take small steps, walk with a careful gait, and have trouble negotiating corners—just like astronauts, though to a lesser extent. Increased sensitivity and tenderness of the soles of the feet is another feature seen in both groups. Many of these symptoms are also common features in the elderly. These problems can have serious consequences when those who suffer from them face such challenges as walking across uneven terrain, negotiating obstacles in their path, operating complex equipment, or driving a car in fast-moving traffic.

When Senator Glenn took part in the 1998 flight on *STS-95*, he and three of his younger fellow crew members (ages thirty-eight to forty-two) took the platform test three times before and four times after the flight. Before the flight, the ability of the seventy-seven-year-old Glenn to control his posture, as shown by the test, was well above average for his age group. After landing, his postural stability was seriously disrupted. But it had fully recovered by the fourth day after his return, and this rate of recovery was similar to that recorded by the younger crew-members.

To improve our understanding of the characteristics of falls in the elderly, the platform test is now being used in the Baltimore Longitudinal Aging Study. This study, run by the National Institute on Aging (NIA), has every two years monitored the health of a large number of people over a period of fifty years. Bill Pal-oski of NASA and Jeffrey Metter of the NIA have been documenting the similarities in changes in balance and postural stability between returning astro-nauts and 280 members of this study as they grow older. The test is very sensitive and is able to pick up even slight changes in balance well before obvious deficits occur in older people. An early warning is of considerable importance, because 40% of the elderly people who need treatment in hospital after a fall die within a year. Every year, more than 200,000 Americans lose their mobility because they suffer hip fractures when they fall. Eventually, scientific comparisons between balance problems experienced by astronauts and those suffered by the elderly are expected to lead to better fall-prevention advice and to an improved quality of life in later years.

What about the Other Senses?

Returning astronauts have mentioned the fact often enough for it to be noteworthy that food does not taste as good in space. It seems much blander. A salt solu-tion drunk before re-entry to expand blood volume, in the hope that it will prevent fainting after landing, is hard to swallow before flight but becomes palat-able in space. Rats in head-down simulation experiments on the effects of space show an increased appetite for salt.

U.S. astronaut Norm Thagard lost 37.4 lbs (17 kg) on his 115-day stay aboard the Russian spacecraft *Mir* in 1995, mostly because of his distaste for the Soviet Space diet, which is rich in fish. Yet he had plenty of time during his long train-ing period to get accustomed to what was coming. What had changed? Is it only the taste buds that are affected in spaceflight, or is it also the sense of smell? Knowing what caused these changes is important to remaining healthy during long stays in space, but taste and smell are also extremely important as we grow older here on Earth in maintaining our appetite for normal nutrition.

Choc Shock for a Space Jock

Astronaut Jim Bagian, an avowed chocoholic, sneaked a precious Mars bar aboard his first Shuttle flight in 1989. Finding a quiet moment to tuck into his secret trove, he was dismayed to discover that he did not experi-ence the pleasurable taste sensation he had been looking forward to. In fact, he admitted, "It tasted foul." The problem, of course, was not with the Mars bar; it was a consequence of the way space had affected the astronaut's taste buds and sense of smell.

People who complain that their food has lost its flavor—and who may, as a consequence, be in danger of becoming malnourished—may actually be losing not their sense of taste but their sense of smell. The taste buds can pick out only four basic sensations: bitter, salty, sour, and sweet. To distinguish a flavor such as chocolate from that of strawberries, the nose and taste buds need to work together.

We do not all taste food the same way. We know that some people are not fazed by very hot, spicy food, whereas others cannot tolerate it. It is believed that one person in four inherits the ability to be a "super taster," and Linda Bastoshuk at Yale University Medical School uses a simple lab test to identify such people. These more sensitive tasters—often women—have more taste buds and tend to be thinner, perhaps because they find that smaller portions are sufficient. By contrast, less sensitive tasters are more likely to seek out very sweet, fatty, or spicy foods. "Making foods more or less attractive to people has tremendous dietary significance," she claims.

When the Taste Buds Go "On Strike"

Jim Weilfenbach, at the National Institute of Dental and Cranial Facial Research, in Bethesda, Maryland, made a study of ninety-one men and seventy-nine women to find whether loss of taste is inevitable with age. His answer was "No." He argued that many things happen to a person over a lifetime that may cause taste problems and that a direct relationship with age cannot be proven. Viral infections, the common cold, clogged sinuses, and dental problems can all affect the senses of taste and smell. Perhaps people with a bad cold should say, "I can't smell anything." But they don't. They say, "I can't taste anything."

It has been known for more than thirty years that changes in the levels of sex hormones and in steroids put out by the adrenal glands affect thresholds of taste, smell, and hearing. These senses are more acute in people who have low levels of adrenal steroids, brought on by some deficiency or disease. Their taste perception is not only greater than that of normal subjects, but it can be one hundred times more accurate. Their hearing is sharper, too. Treatment with the synthetic steroid prednisolone, often used to treat serious allergic reactions and inflammation, has brought back hearing and taste thresholds to normal.

People treated for a long time with steroids for arthritis or allergic conditions may also find they experience some loss in taste and should be aware of these side effects. Similarly, those in highly stressful circumstances, who are producing very high levels of their own adrenal steroids, may also notice reductions in smell, taste, and hearing sensitivity. Some elderly people find themselves in this category, and one way to improve these senses may be to learn how to manage the stress in their lives more effectively. In the meantime, increasing the amount of flavoring in their cooking with herbs and spices should help them to get more enjoyment from their food, and so avoid becoming undernourished.

Must Your Eyesight and Hearing Always Get Worse with Age?

Impaired vision and poor hearing are accepted as part and parcel of getting old. People who have prided themselves on the acuteness of their eyesight can find that they need reading glasses by the time they reach their fifties, or even earlier. Hearing aids are commonplace among the over-seventies. It appears though, that gravity has a part to play in keeping hearing and eyesight up to the mark.

In the early days of the space program, scientists predicted that in conditions of zero gravity, eyeballs might fall out, or at least change in shape. None of this happened. However, an astronaut's visual acuity is certainly reduced after returning from space—especially during walking.

Mir cosmonauts have reported reduced hearing. This has been blamed on the relatively high background noise in their spacecraft from motors and fans, though no systematic measurements have been taken. The Russians have also reported some hearing loss in volunteers lying head-down in bed. Studies of volunteers who have spent 62 to 120 days in bed-rest showed a decrease in the ability to discriminate sounds. However, none of these changes were permanent.

• Touching is Good for the Brain

Not a great deal is known about how the sense of touch changes as we grow older, though we seem to be less ticklish than we were as children. Nevertheless, we do know how important touch is to the normal development of babies. There are many studies showing that if you touch, nurture, and hug babies, there are certain types of structural connections in the brain that become a lot stronger than if you don't. The brains of babies not touched or nurtured end up being 20 to 30% smaller than normal, with all that this implies for later development.

I am not aware of similar studies in the elderly, but many who are in nursing homes find that their opportunities for social interaction are reduced and that they are not often touched in an affectionate and caring way. Significant changes in the skin would also suggest that with advancing years there is less sensitivity to touch. Eddie Longman, my dentist, who has been in practice for more than thirty years, says that his older patients are "ostensibly less sensitive to pain." They will let him work without Novocain on roots and fillings in a way younger people would not tolerate.

What Can You Do about It?

Prevention

Prevention is always better than cure, because once the damage is done it may not be easy to correct. Avoid loud noise, for it can cause hearing loss. Protect your eyes in bright sunlight, for it can cause damage and lead to cataracts. Even *doggles*—sunglasses for dogs—are now available. Maintaining basic health habits goes a long way. Healthy gums and teeth are important to taste and smell. Stroking a pet or a child or hugging a friend or partner helps to stimulate touch receptors.

Technology

Ever-improving hearing aids, glasses, lens implants, and other devices are now available. We have come a long way from the hearing horn that Beethoven had to use. New hearing aids can be surgically implanted in the middle ear instead of sitting in the outer ear. This solves many of the problems that make hearing aids less desirable to some. Today's hearing aids do a good job of helping people hear though they have not yet managed to suppress all background noise. It may sometimes be difficult to distinguish between the echo of a user's own voice, the voice of the person to whom they are talking, and that of another person nearby. About 700 people have the surgical implants in the U.S., and further improvements are bound to develop.

Healthy Eating and Antioxidants

What you eat can have a direct effect on your hearing and eyesight. A build-up of free radicals, caused by pollutants and a poor diet, can damage vision and lead to hearing loss. Jochen Schacht, scientific director of the Kresge Hearing Research Institute at the University of Michigan, studies the causes of hearing loss from noise and from antibiotics such as streptomycin, that are toxic to the hearing system. He finds that if antioxidants such as aspirin are administered with the antibiotic, hearing loss can be prevented. Similarly antioxidant combinations of

Vitamins, A, C and E with zinc and copper and lutein can give protection against free radicals and are now recommended by ophthalmologists for healthy eyes.

Regeneration

One important and promising solution is still in the research stage. The inner ear has thousands of microscopic hair cells, tuned to vibrate in response to different levels and pitches of sound. The loss of these cells as we age is the leading cause of human deafness. Imagine if we could get them to regenerate! The Deafness Research Foundation in Washington, D.C., claims the ability to replenish these cells could end more than 70% of deafness. It could also be effective against tinnitus, the sensation of ringing in the ears that can be caused by hair cell loss.

Until fifteen years ago, the medical world believed that once a hair cell had gone, it had gone forever. Hearing loss was inevitable and irreversible with aging. Then, two separate groups of researchers found that birds spontaneously re-grow damaged hair cells and regain hearing, whereas mammals, including humans, do not. Progress has been slow, but such a discovery has huge potential. One encouraging finding comes from the work of Jeffrey Corwin at the University of Virginia. He found that the hair cells from the vestibular system in the inner ear of mammals, both rats and humans, regenerate just like the hearing hair cells of birds. Though the hair cells for hearing and balance are different, they function in much the same way. It is therefore probable that this discovery will one day make possible regenerative treatments for hearing cells as well.

• The Plastic Brain

The brain is amazingly adaptable. Just like muscle, it even changes structurally to meet new demands. We call this ability to adjust "neural plasticity." NASA scientist Muriel Ross showed that this change happens much more rapidly than previously thought. The number of synapses of the hair cells in the inner ear of rats increased dramatically within twenty-four hours of being in the reduced gravity of space. They were back to normal within twenty-four hours of returning to Earth's gravity after a stay of fourteen days in space.

With every new environment, be it in space or on Earth, the brain needs to readapt. The more often you go back and forth between the same two environments, the faster the brain adapts and readapts. Space travel is one example of this. Another is what happens in the case of scuba divers. At first they have a problem under water judging how far away things are. But with repeated diving, their visual systems adjust instantly as they go in and out of the water. If they do not dive for a long time, they may have to readapt, though this process happens much faster once it is learned. Most sailors get seasick at first but eventually adapt to going back and forth between land and sea. Of course, there are always exceptions. It is said that British hero Admiral Lord Nelson got seasick every time he put to sea.

Pointing at a Target

Moving your arm to point to a target or reach for a particular object is a simple task of coordination. The arm has to move the right distance, at the right speed, while anticipating and compensating for the force of gravity pulling it down. Several control loops in the brain, the eyes, the vestibular system, and the arm are involved in this simple task, which we do many times a day. A baby needs a few trials to get it right for the first time. Some older people may also have a problem reaching for objects with accuracy. They compensate by slowing down the motion to allow their eyes to take on a greater role.

Eye-hand coordination exercises, preferably in the standing position, where the pull of gravity is greatest, both with eyes open and with eyes closed, may help to restore coordination and the perception of gravity. In space, astronauts tend at first to overshoot their target because gravity is no longer pulling their arm down, and it takes a few attempts to get it right. At the opposite end of the gravity scale, by increasing gravity on a centrifuge you would point well below the target, because your arm would be pulled down more than you expected. However, the brain learns quickly.

New Hope for Victims of Spinal-Cord Injury

The spinal cord, an extension of the brain consisting of nerve fibers, neurons, and blood vessels, is more than just a passive conduit shuttling information back and forth to and from the brain. Anton Wernig, in Germany; Serge Rossignol, in Canada; and Reggie Edgerton, in the U.S., have found that spinal-cord neurons are capable of learning. Their research provides some hope for victims of spinal-cord injury. Like neurons in the brain, the spinal neurons change in response to stimuli from the environment and retain the memory of what they have learned. Edgerton and his group at UCLA found that the spinal cord, even when completely separated from the brain, is sensitive to changes in the weight loading of limbs. A UCLA rehabilitation team, led by Susan Harkness, literally trains the spinal cord of patients suffering from this paralyzing injury to enable them to *walk* on a treadmill.

First they are manually helped to place their feet down, one at a time, while they are partially supported in a harness. A prerequisite is that the injury to the spinal cord is at a level low enough to allow the arms, with the help of the harness, to keep the body upright. Practicing the same stepping pattern over and over again, for one and a half hours a day over three to six months, has helped many such patients walk with no more assistance than that of a cane or a walker.

Walking in this case is not what we normally think of as perfectly coordinated locomotion, but it is good enough to allow patients to get out of their wheelchairs and move about. Injury victims with some remaining connections to the brain obviously do best. Those with injury higher up and paralyzed from the neck down, such as *Superman* actor Christopher Reeve, require total support and therefore take longer to achieve results.

Staying Active

Remember some of the things we did as children, like playing hopscotch, skipping rope, or dancing? As we give up such activities with the passing years, the brain circuits act as if they had gone into space, and the old adage "use it or lose it" comes into play. Many things we do every day depend on "standing up" to gravity, to keep our balance and coordination of movements tuned. If we carry on doing them we will have fewer balance problems later on. If we don't, it is never too late to start. So keep dancing—and remember: it takes regular stimulation and a good deal of repetition to keep the brain circuits sharp.

Virtual Reality and Other New Technologies

NASA's Jacob Bloomberg is developing ways to help astronauts preserve their ability to stand and walk when they return to Earth. These depend on new technologies known as virtual reality and augmented reality, and they are similar to those used in computer displays and video games. He and others have found that by using different challenges in combination, you can train the brain to become more adaptable. It turns out that people feel comfortable when looking at pictures with strong vertical images—trees in a landscape or rooms with windows and high-backed chairs. But if you show someone such a scene and then start rotating it, they have a hard time standing upright. Bloomberg uses a screen like that on a laptop computer to display visual patterns, such as a virtual office scene. The visual flow of patterns on the screen is changed to get the brain working in overdrive, stimulating it to adapt to the changing scene.

Similarly, in space, strongly vertical scenes can be projected by means of virtual-reality goggles, which astronauts wear when working out on a treadmill. This exercise is believed to help give the brain strong visual cues that normally couple the sensation of gravity with the activities of walking and running. Such cue reinforcement does not replace gravity, but it may maintain the brain's memory of gravity even though the body does not sense it. It may also enhance the value of the exercise in space, an activity that has not so far proved to be very effective on its own.

Whereas virtual reality is intended to replace the real world, augmented reality adds to the user's sensory perceptions of his world by packing more information into it. Advances in both technologies should make it possible to replace and increase most missing gravity cues necessary to stimulate sensors in the body. Though most advances rely on vision, other senses, such as touch and hearing, can also be augmented with virtual information. Augmented reality systems are being used in the operating theater, in computer games, and by soldiers training for battle. NASA scientists at Ames, in California, were among the first to study such systems, in the 1970s and 1980s. Someday, special video games could also be useful in the rehabilitation of the disabled and the elderly. In space, where gravity cues are almost non-existent, increasing the intensity of visual, touch, or auditory cues may compensate for their absence. In the elderly, or in people with balance disorders, where the sensitivity of the receptors may be reduced but where gravity is present, enhancement of gravity and other sensory stimulation could have a similar beneficial effect.

The Force of Hypergravity

Enhancement of the gravity cues on Earth, the state known as hypergravity, depends on the principle that the faster any mass moves, the heavier it becomes. Jump up and down on a weighing machine and the needle will swing wildly, reaching far beyond the line that indicates your normal weight. Riding a bicycle, speeding in a fast car, riding a roller coaster, flying in a airplane, whizzing down-hill on a sled, or spinning on a centrifuge all provide the stimulation of hyper-gravity. Rocking chairs are objects we usually associate with the elderly, just as we associate cradles with babies. There may be good physiological reasons why human beings at either end of the age spectrum find comfort in the motion of rocking.

Studies of hypergravity on the ground suggest that a short-arm centrifuge onboard a spacecraft could provide intermittent periods of gravity exposure. With the head at the center, the astronaut would be oriented so that maximum gravity would be at his or her feet. This should be most useful in preventing mus-cle and bone loss by weight loading the lower extremities. It would also draw the blood towards the feet, just as in standing, and so stimulate the heart and blood circulation. While lying the other way, with the feet at the center, the head could be positioned so as to concentrate the artificially created gravity on the region of the inner ear. Experiments on a rotating chair on the *Neurolab* Shuttle mission in 1998 suggested that this is indeed a feasible way of stimulating the organs of the inner ear to maintain the sharpness of their gravity sensors. Similar exposure to a force greater than 1G on a centrifuge on Earth might one day prove useful in restoring a sense of balance to elderly people who have lost it.

Exercises anybody can do

Exercises that challenge the sense of balance are by far the best way to maintain it. They set a task not only for the inner ear but also for the ability to coordinate other parts of the body involved in preventing falls. It is always useful in any training program to do a number of different exercises, all designed to have the same end result.

• Tai Chi, Yoga, and Pilates

The ancient art of *tai chi* is practiced to this day in many lands where the Chinese have left their cultural imprint, from the gardens of Hong Kong to the streets of San Francisco. It involves slow, flowing, deliberate, ballet-like movements that require good balance. A 1992 study, using a test of balancing on one leg, found that old persons who practiced *tai chi* did better than those who did not—and, more importantly, they had up to a 50% lower incidence of falls. By contrast, research that tried to reduce falling by means of general exercise training produced mixed results. Other exercises, such as yoga and stretching, can improve flexibility. Yoga also includes many positions that promote good balance.

Strengthening the muscles of the trunk is effective in improving posture and balance, since it strengthens the abdomen, the lower back muscles, and the buttocks. Here again, Pilates exercises, also known as "core training," can be of great benefit. (See Chapter 3, "Flexing Muscle.")

• Standing on One Leg

Balancing on one leg as long as possible and then the other, is the most commonly used test of balance. Simple though it is for most of us, people with foot problems may find it difficult. Another simple way of testing and improving your balance is to see how far you can walk when you place one foot in front of the other, touching heel to toe. If you lose your balance after a few steps, keep doing the exercise every day until you improve. Astronauts test their balance on a posture platform that can sway forward and back, and they do it both with eyes open and with eyes shut. These platforms are now also used clinically. In 1991, a three-year exercise study of older women who maintained an active lifestyle reported they could stand on one leg twice as long as their inactive counterparts.

• Quadruped Balance

With your knees and hands on an exercise mat, extend one arm straight ahead and the opposite leg straight back as far as possible. Keep your hips and shoulders level, head straight ahead, abdominal muscles contracted, and back flat. Hold the position as you count slowly to five. Repeat with the other arm and leg. Begin by doing a set of five on each side. It is more important to focus on the quality of each repetition than on the number of repetitions. When you have the form right, increase the number of sets. To step up the challenge, use two foam half rolls and eventually two foam rolls to support your knees and hands.

• Say Goodbye to Shuffling

Walking becomes more of a shuffle with age or inactivity. Many falls are caused by tripping over one's feet. To improve your gait and avoid shuffling, make an effort when you walk, even around the house, to lift your feet well off the ground and to deliberately place each foot down heel first. You may feel silly doing this, but think of it as an exercise. Improve the mobility of your ankles by gently rocking on your feet back and forth from heel to toe. Then roll your feet to their outer sides and then back to the inner part of the sole. If this is too difficult to do standing up, try sitting in a chair first and then progress to standing. Evaluate your progress by seeing how long you can balance on one foot or how far you can walk heel to toe in a straight line.

Tracking Progress

For a more fun test, take a six-foot roll of brown wrapping paper and lay it on the floor in a corridor or the garage. Get an old pair of tennis shoes and, using heavy marker pens, paint the bottom of one shoe blue and the other red. Put them on and step onto your brown paper. Start walking in what you think is a straight line from one end of the paper to the other. Stop and take your shoes off. With a measuring tape, measure the distance of one or two steps (blue to blue, or red to red), and then measure the width between the left and right foot (the red and blue step). Look at the ink marks on the paper. Are they clean outlines or smudged from shuffling? If you have a grandchild this is a good one to do with them, since you can compare the difference. Are their imprints cleaner than yours, and are they closer together?

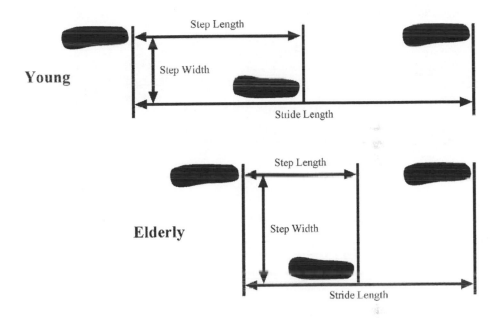

The step length and width in young (above) and old persons (below). Step length becomes shorter and width greater with age. Tracings obtained by walking on brown paper wearing shoes with ink-stained soles. [By permission from G. W. Schmid-Schonbein et al. (eds.), Frontiers in Biomechanics (New York: Springer Verlag, 1986) 226.]

Repeat this test after three to six months of doing these exercises or joining a *tai chi* class. See if you are now walking with your feet closer together, taking longer steps, and not shuffling. Can you walk down a street without looking at your shoes? Can you go down the stairs without looking at your feet? If so, you are on your way to better balance and coordination. As with all other systems in the body, there is plenty of evidence that good balance and coordination depend on how often they are used. As with other systems, it is the number of times an activity is performed, not the duration of the activity, that is most important.

Keeping the Senses Tuned

If your senses are blunted for whatever reason, you become isolated from the world, a prisoner inside a numb body. You may feel that nobody seems to care about you or, if they do, that you cannot see or hear it. Many older citizens feel that way. Is the decline in sensory function inevitable? How can we escape from this prison and regain our freedom? Keeping the senses sharp is critical to our well-being. It is not too hard to stay well balanced and coordinated. Gravity comes to the rescue if only we take care to use it.

5

Why It Is Vital to Keep Changing Posture

○ ○
If one's posture is upright, one has no need to fear a crooked shadow.

—*Chinese proverb*

After only nine hours in space, Wally Schirra, one of America's original seven astronauts, complained of "wooziness" when he tried to stand on the recovery ship's flight deck. That was in October 1962. Since then, 75% of U.S. astronauts have reported feeling faint when they stood up again after returning to Earth. Russian cosmonauts have experienced the problem, and the longer they stay in space, the worse it hits them when they get back to Earth. After missions that have lasted several months, cosmonauts have been put in reclining chairs at the recovery site. Some have fainted even in this position and have been unable to leave the site under their own accord.

It is not just returning astronauts and cosmonauts who suffer from wooziness. You may well know the feeling yourself, for it can affect anybody who stays in bed for as little as a day. Have you ever felt faint and dizzy when you stood up suddenly? Or temporarily lost your balance and almost fallen over? The fact that living in space and lying in bed can give rise to the same symptoms suggests that the root cause is the same in both cases: a reduction in the force of gravity or a change in the way we use it.

As we go about our daily lives, what we do in gravity and the way we orient ourselves towards this downward-pulling force has a direct effect on our state of health. It stimulates many different systems, most of the time without our even being aware of it. Faintness and dizziness, sometimes leading to a fall, can overcome people of any age. Anyone who has stopped exercising because of procrastination, age, or illness will recognize some of these symptoms. However, the consequences of a fall become more serious as we get older.

Sedentary habits—sitting around or lying in bed for much of the day—encourage a tendency to faint on standing, and they are all too easy to pick up. We know from research in space that they lead to a reduction in the muscle mass of the heart and cause the muscle walls of blood vessels to become thinner. As you become less active, you grow more susceptible to heart-rhythm abnormalities, meaning each heart beat becomes less efficient. You'll huff and puff when climbing stairs or working in the garden. Even after a short walk, your heart will pound and you will soon be out of breath and gasping for air.

How the System Works

If you fill a tube-shaped balloon with water and lay it on its side, the water will distribute evenly throughout the balloon. Stand it up and the base will swell as water is pulled down by gravity, leaving a smaller volume at the top. The more water in the balloon and the less stretchy it is, the more rigid it will be and the smaller the difference between the amounts of water at the top and base.

This is pretty much how our circulatory system works—or at least, how it would work if it were not for the fact that we are equipped with a pump called the heart. Lie down and blood is distributed evenly throughout your body. Put your head lower than your feet and blood shifts towards your head and chest, drawn there by gravity. Something very similar happens to astronauts when they go into space, where the force of gravity is virtually zero. When they stand up again back on Earth, blood rushes to their legs and feet, under the force of gravity. Their upper bodies get less blood and their heads may get very little or none.

The heart is the pump, and the blood vessels are the pipelines in a transport system that delivers oxygen and nutrients to all parts of the body, but most importantly to the brain. Blood vessels are elastic, and major vessels such as the arteries can themselves pump the blood along. Veins, which carry the blood back to the heart, have valves that prevent it from flowing backwards. Without these valves and resilient, elastic vein walls, the blood would flow back to swell the feet and legs, when you sit or stand up. Just like an old, well-used piece of elastic, the vein walls over-stretch with time, losing their elasticity and allowing the blood to pool in the feet.

A Tip from the Guards at Buckingham Palace

If you had to stand still for hours at a time, you might literally become light-headed, despite all the body's ingenious mechanisms for supplying blood to the head. This is because gravity is working all the time to pull blood from your head into your lower body and legs. If you contract your muscles, as you do when you exercise, they squeeze the blood upward in the veins they surround. But if you are standing still, the heart cannot call on any such support.

The guardsmen who stand motionless on sentry duty outside Buckingham Palace have worked out a way to overcome the problem. From time to time, unknown to the spectators, they contract their calf muscles. This squeezes blood vessels in the legs and pushes more blood upwards. If they did not do this, guards would run the risk of fainting on duty.

What Happens When You Stand Up?

Standing up, which appears on the surface to be one of the simplest of all physical actions, is far from simple when you consider the complex responses it sets in motion. First, gravity causes blood and other fluids to shift away from the head to the lower body and legs. The result is that you will register a different blood pressure in different parts of your body—what doctors call a pressure gradient. The pressure at your head, for instance, may be 70 mm Hg (mercury). At your heart it will be 100 mm Hg and at your feet as high as 200 mm Hg.

Pressure and volume sensors in your neck and chest read this as a danger signal. They interpret it to mean that there is less blood volume in the whole body. They flash neural, hormonal, and chemical messages to your heart and kidneys to respond to the threat. The heart beats faster, and each beat pushes out more blood than before. In order to expand your blood volume, your kidneys cut down on the loss of water and salt by putting out less urine. In this way, blood volume and pressure are maintained and sufficient blood continues to flow to your head.

Continuous standing calls further protective measures into play. For example, fluid from the surrounding tissues is pulled into the bloodstream, expanding the total volume of blood in circulation. This expanded volume keeps the blood vessels distended and provides the heart with sufficient volume to pump effectively.

If greater stress than just standing—merely taking a few steps will do it—is put on the body, the heart rate increases further, and even more so after inactivity. But just standing still is a greater challenge than walking with respect to the amount of blood the heart pumps out. This is because standing without moving your leg muscles stimulates constriction of blood vessels and vein stiffness to enable them to resist sudden increases in leg volume the next time you need to stand.

What Happens When You Lie Down?

What happens to the circulation when you lie down is the reverse of what happens when you stand. Blood volume shifts from the legs to the head and chest. When blood shifts upward—as a result of lying down, going into space, or immersing yourself in a pool, where the force of gravity is reduced by the water—the pressure and volume sensors in the neck and chest detect a larger volume. They read this as an increase in the entire body's blood volume and orchestrate a reduction, first and foremost by increasing the amount of urine you put out. This urge to urinate when lying down at night does not happen in healthy people and they are able to sleep uninterrupted.

It is these gravity-powered shifts in volume between the lower and upper parts of the body that occur every time you change posture on Earth that tune the sensors regulating blood pressure. This tuning process is, in effect, switched off when astronauts are in space. Even though they are moving about in the spacecraft, without gravity they have no sensation of standing up or lying down. After the initial response to the rush of blood upward in space, the blood-pressure gradient is eliminated, becoming equal (100 mm Hg) throughout the body.

Lose Your Wrinkles in Space

Astronauts have been described as moon-faced when they are in space, because in the near-total absence of gravity blood rises to their heads, making their faces puffy. One effect of this puffiness is that wrinkles disappear. In fact, just like after a Botox treatment, their faces become somewhat expressionless. Unfortunately, back on Earth the wrinkles return, just as they do when Botox wears off.

Why Don't Giraffes Faint?

There is much we learn from nature. During the course of evolution, other living creatures have developed ingenious ways of maintaining blood pressure at the right level, especially in the head. The giraffe's heart needs to pump very hard to send blood up to its brain at the end of that long neck. You would think giraffes might faint when they raise their heads after drinking, but they don't. They have developed a tough sheath that surrounds their leg muscles, something like internal support hose, that prevents blood from pooling in their leg veins.

According to their habitat, snakes have evolved in various ways to make sure blood gets to the brain. Harvey Littlewood at the University of Florida studies anatomical differences between snakes that live on land, on trees, and in water. Among those that climb trees, the heart is nearest the head, so blood has a shorter distance to travel. In land snakes, the heart is located further down, and in water snakes it is even lower, in the middle of their body. If you were to place a water snake on a tree, it would faint and fall off because of the longer distance blood has to travel to reach its head!

What Can Go Wrong?

Why Do People Faint?

When the body's response mechanisms to the pull of gravity are inadequate, the result is fainting—a slowing of the heart, nausea, pallor, dizziness, and a sudden drop in blood pressure, resulting in a "blackout" when not enough blood flows to the head. The brain is starved of oxygen and a temporary loss of consciousness follows. When people faint, they fall down. This is nature's way of getting blood back to the head so that they can recover consciousness. Tall, lean people are more prone to fainting than short people. In general, women are more susceptible to fainting than men. The reasons are not yet understood, but they seem to involve hormones.

The main purpose of the circulation is to transport to the brain the oxygen we breathe in through the lungs. The circulation must deliver an adequate supply of blood—not too much and not too little—to all parts of the body, but most importantly to the head. In people with high blood pressure, too much blood reaches the head and the result can be a pounding in the head, mental confusion and, in extreme cases, stroke. If your brain gets too little blood, it will be starved of oxygen and energy-generating glucose. At the very least you feel hazy, mental function slows down, or you pass out. If your brain gets no blood at all, it stops working. And if it shuts down for too long, you go into a coma—or die.

Abnormally low blood pressure, injury, and disease can all cause wooziness and fainting. It can also be brought on by antihistamines in cold medications and drugs taken for high blood pressure or other conditions, such as Parkinson's disease. Blood flow to the brain can be reduced after a meal, when it is diverted to the stomach to aid digestion. But the most obvious and common cause of reduced blood volume is dehydration. This can be brought on in many ways.

Water Matters

Donating blood, sunbathing for too long, hot weather, fever, sweating in a sauna, drinking alcohol, dieting, malnutrition, use of diuretics, and simply not drinking enough water can all bring on fainting spells. So can anything that increases the output of urine and reduces blood volume. For example, diabetics may be more prone to fainting because the illness increases the amount of urine they put out. If you are not used to living at a high altitude, going into the mountains can bring on fainting, because the higher you climb, the "thinner" the air becomes—that is, the less oxygen it holds.

Anybody who spends a fair length of time in water may also experience fainting, because water reduces the pull of gravity. The heart does not have to work as hard to pump blood up to the head, and the swimmer may faint when he or she gets out. Swimmers may faint when they get out of a pool—especially if their blood pressure is low—if the water is warm or if it is just a hot day. At a spa in New Mexico, I fainted in my birthday suit as I stepped out of a Jacuzzi after fifteen minutes. Most swimming clubs in the U.S. get children out of the pool for ten minutes every hour as a safety precaution.

The Swimming Pool Syndrome

It is one of the laws of physics that a floating body displaces its own weight. When swimming we become, in effect, weightless. The blood, which on land is pulled down by gravity towards the feet, shifts upwards into the head and chest. Blood-pressure sensors in the head and neck register this as an increase in the amount of liquid in the body and set in motion mechanisms to bring it back down to normal. The fastest way to do this is to get rid of urine, and this is why children and adults alike feel the urge to urinate soon after going into a swimming pool. Adults, of course, feel greater social pressure than children not to do so and are thus more likely to control this urge. Even so, chlorine is pumped into public swimming pools as a general precaution.

The Case for Salt

In the past few decades, nutritionists have focused on curbing the amount of salt in the nation's daily diet. Too much salt causes fluid retention, increases the workload on the kidneys, the heart, and the circulatory system, and so creates the risk of high blood pressure, strokes, and heart disease. Some people with a predisposition to high blood pressure are supersensitive to salt. For them, even average salt intake can raise blood pressure further. They are therefore prescribed diuretics and a low-salt diet to keep their pressure in check and shed retained fluids that produce swollen ankles and a distended abdomen.

In my studies of healthy humans in bed-rest, regulating salt intake was crucial to the accuracy of the results. My awareness of what constitutes "normal salt intake" became much sharper, particularly in our collaborations with other countries. In the 1970s, our Shuttle diet contained 5 g salt per day. During our joint studies with the Germans and the Soviets, I was amazed to find out that they considered this level "low." At the time, the average salt intake in Germany was 8 g/day and in the Soviet Union it was 15 g/day.

The anti-salt campaign has been a marked success. The average salt intake in the U.S. since the 1980s has been halved from 5 g/day to 2.5 g/day, and many "salt-free" products are now on the market. But for some it can also be harmful to go to the other extreme, to eat too little salt. Salt plays a key role in regulating the fluid balance of the body. Just as too much salt causes a build-up of fluids in the body, so eating too little stimulates the body to get rid of water by passing more urine. Many rapid weight-loss diets depend on this principle. If you follow a low-salt diet—considerably lower than 2.5 g/day—when you don't really need to, this can lead to dehydration, causing you to faint when you stand up. This is certainly not desirable in astronauts or in elderly people who do not suffer from high blood pressure.

The Skin Stores Salt

An important discovery from research in space and bed-rest studies is the capacity of skin to store salt. This salt is stored in an inactive form. When first going into space or lying head-down in bed, humans lose water and salt in the urine until the body equilibrates to the new lower blood volume. Water balance (what is taken in minus what is excreted) returns to normal, but, paradoxically, salt is increasingly retained. German scientists Rupert Gerzer and Martina Heer at the Flight Research Institute (DLR), in Cologne, measured these changes over 120 days in space in the Russian cosmonaut Manarov. They calculated that the amount of salt he stored reached levels that would have normally required him to retain another 8 liters of water, causing very serious edema. But this did not happen.

Where was all this salt going, and why was water not being retained? It was not until some years later that another group of scientists at the University of Berlin found in rat studies that all of the salt retained was contained only in the skin. Biopsies of skin in volunteers during bed-rest showed a similar increase in stored salt. Returning to a normal active state reduced this salt store.

Rats who are genetically predisposed to high blood pressure are unable to store excess salt in their skin. It is anticipated that persons with high blood pressure will show a similar defect in this salt-storing mechanism. We do not yet know where and how such large amounts of salt can be stored in the skin in an apparently inactive form and what purpose they might serve. It does appear to be a gravity- and activity-dependent mechanism with important implications for those who suffer from high blood pressure as well as swollen feet and abdomens.

The Fainting Astronaut

In space, where circulation does not have to cope with gravity, the heart chambers and blood vessels in the head and chest are initially stretched by an inrush of blood. Volume sensors in the carotid artery in the neck and in the upper chamber of the heart initiate the process of bringing it back to what is "normal" for the new gravity-free environment. They send out a host of nerve impulses and hormone signals with the ultimate purpose of reducing the total blood volume.

During the first three or four days in space, more than half of all astronauts experience some form of space sickness, including a general feeling of un-wellness, stomach awareness, loss of thirst and appetite, nausea, and vomiting. These symptoms are clearly linked to the vestibular system of the inner ear, the system that controls balance.

Female astronauts are more susceptible to fainting when they stand up after spaceflight than their male counterparts. This is because they tend to have a higher heart rate and their blood vessels are less able to expand and constrict than those of men. Add to that the reduced blood volume when they return from space, so their hearts pump out less blood with each stroke, and they are more likely to faint.

Older people, by contrast, are usually better able to maintain blood pressure after spaceflight or bed-rest. This is believed to be because their arteries have become stiffer with age. Their tendency towards higher blood pressure turns out to be an asset in this case. In tests on a centrifuge designed to simulate the Gaccelerations generated during re-entry on the Space Shuttle, men aged fifty-five to sixty-five have tolerated high G-forces better than twenty-five to thirty-five-year-old volunteers. On his return after nine days in space, seventy-seven-year-old John Glenn's heart was pumping more efficiently than that of younger men, and his blood pressure was adequately high when he landed.

Fainting immediately after landing has been a serious problem for returning astronauts for more than forty years, and so far no effective solution has been discovered. It could, just like space sickness, become a problem for any future space tourist. But progress has been made. Several potential solutions, including drugs, gravity or hypergravity on the spacecraft by means of a centrifuge, and an inflated G-suit developed by the Air Force worn during re-entry and landing, are being evaluated. These remedies can be useful in earthlings who suffer from similar fainting spells.

The Cult of the Victorian Chaise Lounge

Victorian literature and art are full of images of pale, languid women reclining on red velvet upholstered chaise lounges and fanning themselves, attended by maids. It was fashionable in some classes of society to swoon at the slightest physical or emotional exertion, and the wearing of tight corsets increased women's propensity to faint by interfering with the free flow of blood. They needed attendants around them, because they were so debilitated that they could not take care of themselves—a dire warning of the dangers of inactivity.

Standing Up Is Good for You

Going into space is the extreme way of removing the gravity stimulus that standing up and frequent posture changes usually provide. The result: fainting, wooziness, and problems with blood pressure. Staying in bed, or generally being sedentary and inactive, will produce the same effect. It may take longer, but the result will be the same. Even prolonged sitting produces the same effect. Studies done forty years ago in volunteers who were asked to sit in a chair for three days showed that they too had a tendency to faint on standing up.

The bottom line is that you are most prone to fainting if you live a life in which, by choice or by accident, your response systems are not stimulated often enough by changes in posture many times throughout the day.

How Big Is Your Heart?

The heart of an astronaut, as measured by ultrasound or echocardiography, gets smaller in space. Continuous bed-rest down here on Earth produces similar results. Under both conditions the heart gets smaller, because after an initial upward shift of blood, the volume of blood in the heart is reduced. This is because without gravity, the body's total blood volume adjusts at 10–15% lower than on Earth. This in turn reduces the pumping demands on the heart, and, like any other muscle, when it has less work to do it diminishes in size. Changes in the heart muscle wall, called *cardiomyopathy*, predispose the heart to arrhythmias. Both the size of the heart muscle cells and their number are reduced after longer stays in space.

Heart size increases again when astronauts return to Earth or after people get out of bed and resume normal activity, but it can take a long time. For every day in space, it takes at least one day of recovery, even with the most careful rehabilitation program. In space, the heart also shifts upwards in the chest cavity, since it is not being pulled down by gravity, but it moves down again once back on Earth.

The performance of the heart is affected not only by its size but also by its mechanical properties. The stiffness of the heart muscle determines how well it stores and uses energy as it beats. The heart muscle of anybody who lies in bed longer than thirty days will lose stiffness, and a limp heart is a less efficient pump.

It also becomes more susceptible to arrhythmia—an irregular heartbeat. This can become a life-threatening condition, for it means that the heart is fluttering rather than pumping blood out in synchronized, efficient contractions. The only space mission so far that has been aborted happened in 1987, when Soviet cosmonaut Aleksandr Laveikin, aboard *Mir*, experienced cardiac arrhythmia while working outside the spacecraft. He had to be brought back to Earth. Arrhythmia induced by exertion is not uncommon in athletes, but it is transient and not usually regarded as indicative of a serious problem.

Are Your Pipelines Elastic?

It is not only the heart muscle that can change. Blood vessels also respond to a smaller blood volume. It has been suggested that in response to this reduced blood volume in space, arteries constrict to keep the blood flowing and they no longer see the shear forces that stimulate arterial walls.

When an astronaut finally returns to Earth or when volunteers stand up after a period in bed, the bulk of the blood goes down to their lower legs and the blood vessels are unable to constrict further. Less blood reaches the heart, which is unable to pump out enough blood. Blood pressure falls. Less blood flows to the head, bringing on fainting.

Michael Delp at Texas A&M University is eager to study rats in space to confirm the dramatic thinning and weakening of blood vessel walls that he observed in rats in his lab. These rats had been deconditioned by lifting the load of their bodies off their hind limbs. He explains that just as in other muscles that are underused, the muscle walls of these blood vessels become thinner and weaker when there is a reduction in the pressure changes and chemical signals that normally keep them responsive.

This laboratory research, along with the findings in astronauts, is relevant to anybody, young or old, who leads a sedentary lifestyle or spends a significant amount of time in bed.

Getting Out Of Shape

Deconditioning is a term that describes what happens to a body that is out of shape, or not in its best form. In space, this comes about fairly quickly. On Earth, decreased blood volume, muscle weakness, reduced ability to exercise, and fainting when standing up are all features of deconditioning.

Normally, the body contains about 5 liters (8.8 pints) of blood. More than half of this volume, the fluid portion, is plasma, and the rest is made up of red and white blood cells and platelets. Plasma volume in the blood of astronauts is reduced by 8–10% in the first two or three days in space. It continues to decrease for two to four weeks, until it stabilizes at about 15–20% less than what it was before going into space. On Earth, a 30% reduction in plasma volume has been measured in bed-rest studies of 100–200 days, suggesting a continued slow loss.

As plasma volume decreases, the cell portion of the blood, the hematocrit, appears proportionally greater. However, after two weeks, astronauts on the Skylab missions in 1973 had 15% fewer red blood cells. The red cells contain the oxygen-carrying protein hemoglobin, so a reduction in their number reduces the capacity of blood to deliver oxygen to where it is needed. Changes in hemoglobin are progressive. Some astronauts have lost as much as 24% in as little as thirty days in space.

Spaceflight has also been shown to reduce levels of the hormone that stimulates the production of red blood cells by the bone marrow. This hormone, called erythropoietin, is known to track athletes and Tour de France cyclists as the blood booster EPO and has been illicitly used by some to enhance their performance. Its use is often referred to as "blood doping." During spaceflight, the red cell mass eventually returns to a level that is normal for the lower plasma volume but still low compared with what it was on Earth. When astronauts get back to Earth, it takes at least sixty days for their number of red cells to return to normal. Anemia in older people has been attributed to poor nutrition, but inactivity, which amounts to not using gravity properly, may also make its contribution.

Don't Lie in Bed Too Long after a Heart Attack

Bed-rest or lack of activity will prolong the time it takes to recover from illness. Patients recovering from a heart attack due to myocardial infarction (death of heart muscle tissue) tire easily and find it hard to exercise. But it is difficult to say to what extent the problem is a result of damage to the heart versus their deconditioning due to lying in bed.

A study by DeBusk and his group at Stanford University showed that one's intolerance to standing and tendency to faint does not depend on the extent to which that person's heart was damaged after a myocardial infarction but on how long he or she had remained in bed after surgery. Their deconditioned state demanded more work and more pumping of oxygen from a less efficient heart muscle. This could be hazardous to those with restricted blood flow. These findings led to the use of low-level supine or upright exercise training in myocardial patients to improve their diminished oxygen transport.

Keeping Your Sensors Tuned

Blood-pressure and volume sensors in the arteries of the neck that regulate the blood-pressure reflex become less responsive with age. Vic Convertino at the U.S. Army Institute of Surgical Research, in Texas, and Dwayne Eckberg at the University of Virginia measured the sensitivity of this reflex. This mechanism initiates the appropriate response when the blood pressure exceeds its normal range. Remarkably, just as in the elderly, they found it had become less sensitive to such changes in thirty-year-old men after only twelve days of bed-rest. Eckberg had measured similarly reduced sensitivity in astronauts after as little as five days in space.

Such reduced sensitivity of the sensors compromises the ability to stand up without fainting. Measurements in those over seventy show that their response to standing is like that of returning astronauts or young adults after a few days of bed-rest. Their hearts beat faster and faster as they try to handle the effort. If they do not succeed, they faint. Like other symptoms common to aging and returning astronauts, this too is reversible by effectively using the stimulus of gravity.

The response of an active, healthy person to standing begins with the sympathetic nerves releasing the chemical transmitter norepinephrine. This causes the arteries to constrict and increases the performance of the heart, sending blood pressure up to maintain adequate circulation.

An inadequate response of the heart and blood vessels after spaceflight or after a period of inactivity was once assumed to be due to reduced sensitivity of the sympathetic nerves which as a result would put out less norepinephrine. In 1998, however, scientists had the opportunity to test this hypothesis on the *Neurolab/STS-90* mission. David Robertson from Vanderbilt University, in Nashville, Gunnar Blomquist from Southwestern University, in Texas, and Eckberg joined forces to prove their theory. They taught the astronauts how to insert a thin wire into the sympathetic nerve in the leg of a fellow astronaut to measure its electrical activity while they were in space. The scientists were anxiously waiting on the ground to measure reduced nerve activity, but the opposite occurred. Fourteen days into the flight, the nerve responded with a normal burst of electrical activity and the blood level of norepinephrine had increased.

We saw similar results in healthy bed-rest volunteers on the ground. The extra norepinephrine is less effective in maintaining blood pressure while standing, because the blood vessels have become less sensitive to it. The result is fainting. Again the message is simple—pressure sensors and blood vessels must be kept responsive. On Earth, the most effective way to do that is to stand frequently. In space, a gravity stimulus must be provided. This can be achieved either by installing an onboard centrifuge or by rotating the spacecraft. Alternatively, it may be possible to fool the body by some other means that, like gravity, induces a shift of blood to the feet. Lower body negative pressure, created by vacuum suction in a box or bag surrounding the body from the waist down, can be used to pull the blood into the lower body.

Keeping All Your Systems Alert

Less stimulation in space, during bed-rest, or aging reduces the responsiveness to other hormones as well. Angiotensin is one of these. In the 1960s, John Luetscher at Stanford University developed ways of measuring the hormone in the blood. Patients with a form of high blood pressure known as "essential hypertension" showed very high systolic blood pressure (the higher reading) and angiotensin in their blood. But when the patients were hospitalized, their blood pressure came back down to normal very quickly. It was concluded that this type of high blood pressure was due to stress and anxiety. Nevertheless, Luetscher's measurements showed that their angiotensin blood levels remained high. He wondered whether lying in bed when hospitalized had anything to do with these paradoxical observations. In a study in young, healthy people confined to bed, Luetscher found that angiotensin blood levels increased after as little as twenty-four hours without any concomitant increase in blood pressure. Many years later, when synthetic angiotensin II became available, we were able to show that its infusion into healthy persons was half as effective in raising blood pressure within ten days of bed-rest. This is another example of some drugs having a much lesser effect in inactive people.

Does Climbing the Stairs Make You Huff and Puff?

The deconditioning that occurs in healthy persons during spaceflight or bed-rest is the body's way of adapting to lower energy requirements. This leads to a reduction in aerobic capacity. With less oxygen, the power of each heartbeat is reduced and the heart must beat faster during exercise to keep up. Muscles that are not used soon become less able to do physical work. An athlete who has been injured and has to give up training for, say, eight weeks will recognize the feeling. So will older people who have given up or cut down on their level of activity.

Maximal oxygen uptake—the volume of oxygen taken in during a maximum bout of exercise—and the capacity for physical work are greater in men than in women, but they decrease in both sexes with age. Tests designed to understand the reasons for this age-related decline suggest that what happens to the elderly is essentially the same as what happens to their younger counterparts as a result of the total inactivity of bed-rest or a flight in the near-zero gravity of space. It just takes longer to develop with age, since presumably people do not give up an active lifestyle all at once but do so over the years.

During exercise, the heart rate increases. As with standing, this response is more marked after a period of inactivity. Most of us are familiar with exercise on a treadmill, used as a standard stress test during an annual physical. As well as measuring how efficiently your heart responds to exertion, the test also measures aerobic capacity—the amount of oxygen consumed during a bout of exercise.

Physical Stress Needs Gravity

Aerobic capacity can be maintained during bed-rest with as little as thirty minutes of horizontal bicycling a day. But this does not prevent the tendency to faint when the bed-rest volunteers later stand. In other words, for aerobic exercise on volume and pressure sensors to have their full benefit, gravity is required.

In space, astronauts are provided with a stationary bicycle or a space treadmill to maintain aerobic fitness. Not all are conscientious about exercising on the treadmill, but the attending flight surgeons can tell who is telling fibs. Some come back with calluses on their soles and others with "baby feet." Shannon Lucid had the best calluses.

Astronaut Steve Hawley, a veteran of five Space Shuttle flights from 1984 to 1999, told me that when he ended a session of pedaling as hard as he could on the bicycle in space, he was surprised to discover that he suddenly felt as if he had not exerted himself at all. This is unlike the sense of exhaustion you would feel after exercising on Earth. We do not understand why this is so.

Fainting When You Stand Can Be a Disease

About half a million people in the U.S. have been documented as suffering from a condition known as pathological *orthostatic hypotension* (OH: the drop in blood pressure when standing), and there may be many more who have the disease but have not been diagnosed. Sufferers find themselves unable to maintain adequate blood pressure upon standing because of genetic or other diseases. Karen Deal, music director and conductor of the Illinois Symphony Orchestra and the Illinois Chamber Orchestra, is one such person. She has been described as "passionate and exuberant." She sits on a stool and conducts with panache. If she stood up to conduct, she would faint and fall over. Many more than the half-million documented cases probably exist.

Physicians are trained to look out for high blood pressure, but they often overlook its opposite—low blood pressure. Anyone who feels light headed in the morning, or when standing in a line on a hot day, may get irritated, as I do, when the nurse taking a blood-pressure reading exclaims how wonderful it is because it is so low. Compared to the debilitating and fatal consequences of high blood pressure, low blood pressure is considered a blessing by medical practitioners. But OH is an illness, too. It can be life threatening, often go undiagnosed, and not receive the attention it deserves.

Being Paralyzed Does Not Mean You Stop Being Active

Paraplegics, those paralyzed by spinal-cord injury, have trouble maintaining their blood pressure when they are helped to sit up. They also suffer from OH. Rick Hansen, the "Man in Motion" Canadian, is a paraplegic who was paralyzed in an accident when he was fifteen years old. Yet he wheeled himself 25,000 miles (40,000 km) around the world from 1985 to 1987. After eight weeks of recovery from his injury, he recalls being put into a recliner bed and brought up slowly, with a warning that "you'll pass out here—everybody does!" In fact he did not, probably through sheer determination.

Once believed to be caused by the spinal injury, OH in paraplegics has now been shown to be preventable by decreasing the amount of time spent lying down, changing posture often (with the help of others), and actually increasing overall activity through upper-body exercises, where at all possible. This is not to say that the lack of nerve stimulation to the legs is not important. Patients who get spinal anesthesia, which temporarily knocks out nerve activity below the point of injection, also invariably show OH when they are first helped up after their surgery.

It is now almost commonplace to see paraplegics whirling their more agile, cambered wheelchairs around the tennis or basketball court or on the dance floor. We have marveled at how wheelchair athletes race each other in marathons. In fact, getting any patient out of bed and out of the hospital is not only good for the health-insurance industry, but is best for the patient's recovery as well.

The Economy Class Syndrome

A well-publicized example of the consequences of inactivity is the incidence of deep-vein blood clots, or thrombosis. It has been called the "economy class syndrome," because it is associated with air travel. It is also associated with being bedridden due to illness. In our bed-rest studies with 167 healthy men and women ranging from nineteen to sixty-five years of age, no incidence of thrombosis was seen. In fact, other researchers have observed the opposite—an increase in the clot-dissolving activity of the blood during bed-rest—especially in women.

Recent studies of the incidence of venous thrombosis during or soon after air travel have pointed to the conclusion that the majority of these incidents occur among those with identifiable risk factors for the formation of blood clots. Whether one is at risk or not, it is a good idea to get up and move about as often as possible during a flight. Drinking plenty of water, not wearing tight clothes, and avoiding leg crossing are also advisable. A stocking that provides mild electrical stimulation to the leg throughout the flight has been reported as helpful in the case of older people who have experienced deep-vein thrombosis on other occasions.

What Can You Do about It?

The incapacitating symptoms brought on by bed-rest or advancing age, which are so much like those we see in space, are the body's way of adapting to the lower demands placed upon it. They are not part and parcel of aging, since they can be reversed. They can certainly be prevented by making very simple lifestyle adjustments. It is not a smart choice to forego the stimulus gravity provides and choose a sedentary lifestyle instead.

The ordinary everyday action of standing up is good for our health. Frequent standing keeps all systems that prevent us from fainting well tuned and in a condition of readiness. It helps keep the heart, blood vessels, and pressure and volume sensors responsive and the circulation in good order so that adequate oxygen-rich blood can always flow through the brain. Avoiding dehydration is crucial to maintain good blood volume. Activities to increase the intake of oxygen, such as aerobic exercise in a gym or other physical exertion that makes us pant for breath, complete the trio of requirements to keep the blood pressure and heart operating within a normal range.

Don't Be a Gravity Dodger!

The easiest way to compromise the response to standing is not to stand. This may sound glaringly obvious, but it is so evident that it is sometimes forgotten. My research has shown that it is the frequency of standing that helps most, not its duration.

But a reduction in the number of times one changes posture can have many causes apart from aging. Some people sit for hours in front of a computer, only to go straight to the TV set and then to bed. This can happen with children and college students just as easily as with the middle-aged or elderly. Whether they know it or not, they have turned into "gravity dodgers."

Lying continuously in bed, of course, reduces the frequency of changes in posture to its lowest possible level. Rolling over in bed does not count as changing posture, because it does not stimulate blood volume or pressure sensors. Only realignment with respect to gravity, such as when you sit or stand up, does that. My point is that the health of the heart and of the entire circulatory system are directly related to how often you stand up every day—how many times you benefit from the full impact of gravity.

Which Matters Most: How Long I Stand or How Often?

For somebody who is prone to fainting, the best long-term cure is to stand up often. This is the best way of using gravity. Simply remaining standing for a long time is not a good thing. The body needs frequent posture changes that alter the column of blood that runs up and down the human body, forcing the sensors, heart, and blood vessels to respond.

The Benefits of Simply Standing

Using gravity to challenge your body keeps the sensors for blood pressure and volume fully primed. If you lead an active and busy life, there will be many occasions during the day when you need to stand up. But those who are less busy have to make their own opportunities. My research has shown that someone who is in bed all the time needs to stand from a lying to an upright position at least eight to sixteen times throughout the day, and preferably more. Many more times will be needed if all you can do is sit up. For those who are bedridden, even raising the head and lowering the foot of the bed or dangling the feet over the side of the bed several times a day can help. Though this will not help prevent bone or muscle loss, it can help prevent falls from fainting.

For those who are not bedridden but are in a nursing home, being helped out of bed for a daily stroll with a walker apparatus and then sitting the rest of the time is not enough. It is better than nothing, but it clearly does not approach the eight or more times of maximal posture change needed.

Getting Blood to Your Head

The importance of providing good circulation to the brain and spinal cord cannot be overestimated. If the brain is not nourished, the rest of the body will not work well either. The simplest way to get blood to your brain is to put your head down. However, bending over is only partially effective. Lying on a bed or on the floor with your knees or legs drawn up, at a level higher than the head for several minutes once a day, is ideal.

As children, my friends and I used to lie on our beds, head hanging down over the end, reading a book or playing board games. I am sure you did it too. Without knowing it, we were nourishing our brains as well as our minds. One of the more advanced yoga positions, and one that is reputed to have significant health benefits, is standing on your head. World-famous violinist Yehudi Menuhin and India's first Prime Minister, Pandit Nehru, were said to carry on great philosophical discussions in this position. Other simpler yoga routines also include positions with the legs up and the head down.

You may also have heard of a device called the Cuban Boots, which became popular a few years ago for achieving in a passive way the same benefits as standing on your head. It consists of a pair of boots attached to a crossbar. Wearing the boots, you can be suspended upside down.

A neighbor of mine spends twenty minutes each day sliding over the back and seat of his armchair until his head is down, legs resting on the seat and supported by his elbows on the floor to read his paper. He claims this helps him think more clearly and that he would not feel right if he missed a day.

Lying head down is not recommended for those with glaucoma—a disease which increases pressure in the eyes—or for those with high blood pressure. If you want to try it, always check with your physician first. Make sure you start slowly, staying down at first for only a few minutes and stopping when you feel uncomfortable, and then gradually increase the time. Always get up slowly, because you may feel faint at first.

Getting Blood to Where It Is Needed

Getting blood to the site of some injuries promotes rapid healing. Sixty-year-old General Hugh Shelton, former chairman of the Joint Chiefs of Staff under President Clinton, fell off a ladder shortly after his retirement. He suffered severe injury and damaged several bones in the back of his neck. His spinal column was not fractured, but compression and inflammation of the spinal cord resulted in paralysis of the arms and legs.

The doctors at the Walter Reed Army Medical Center in Washington, D.C., proposed a new treatment that involved raising his blood pressure, with the drug neosynephrine, and keeping it high for two or three days. A man of his age would normally be at risk of a stroke or heart failure, but because he enjoyed excellent health the doctors went ahead with this innovative treatment. As Shelton's blood pressure was raised, there were signs of slight movement in his arms and legs. This alerted him to the importance of getting as much blood as possible to his upper body. His own determination and the strength training of the rehabilitation program enabled him to make a good recovery, although his right side is still somewhat weak.

Work till You Sweat

In addition to frequent standing, you need to do some aerobic exercise if you can. As long as it is strenuous enough that you work up a sweat and feel short of breath, it will provide a different kind of benefit: it will increase your consumption of oxygen and improve cardiovascular fitness. Aerobic exercise increases cardiac output and stroke volume and increases blood volume, the opposite of what time spent in space or inactive do.

It was once believed that maximum oxygen consumption during exercise—the measure of aerobic fitness—diminished after 25 at the rate of 10% per decade of age. However, oxygen consumption levels have nothing to do with age. A number of more recent studies have shown this decline does not occur among older people who are highly active and do some aerobic exercise, such as walking, bicycling, running, rowing, or stair-climbing. Those who did best were those who started in their early twenties and made aerobic exercise a lifetime habit. But it is never too late to start!

How Much Exercise Is Needed and How Often Should It Be Done?

JoAnn Manson and her colleagues at Brigham and Women's Hospital, in Boston, found that women who walked briskly at least three hours a week or did some more vigorous exercise for a total of one and a half hours a week were 30 to 40% less likely to get coronary heart disease. Along the same lines, a study of 21,000 male physicians who exercised enough to sweat, but only once a week, found that their risk of Type-2 diabetes was reduced by 24%. Stepping up the exercise to two to four times a week reduced their risk by 39%. Sweating is a good indicator of the effectiveness of this type of exercise.

Aerobic exercise is now being found to improve brain power, help those who are depressed, decrease the risk of Type-2 diabetes, and increase good cholesterol, keeping addition to keeping the heart healthy. What's more, studies at Stanford University, in California, now show that one does not need to set aside a big block of time for aerobic exercise to be effective. Three segments of ten minutes each throughout the day were found to be as effective as thirty minutes once a day. Other studies have even found that several segments of as little as eight minutes each were just as effective.

Walk, Swim, or Bike

Treadmill walking uphill for thirty-five to forty minutes a day for six months has been found to be highly beneficial for sixty to eighty-two-year-olds. But a treadmill can be hard on the ankles, knees, and hips of some individuals. Alternative options that have gained popularity are walking, bicycling, swimming, and going up and down the stairs—as long as these activities are done vigorously. Any routine of exercise three times a week that raises the heart rate to somewhere between 70% and 85% of the maximum it would reach with full-out effort is adequate. This is known as the target heart rate (THR), and on average, is said to decrease with age.

The maximum heart rate, which one should never exceed, is around 180 beats a minute for a healthy forty-year-old. This falls by 10 bpm for each decade over that. Therefore, for an eighty-year-old, for example, the maximum is 140. Before starting a new exercise regime, especially if you have been inactive for any length of time, it is always advisable to check with your doctor. If you have a history of heart disease, this is essential. The figures in the table below (Table 5.1) are those recommended by NASA and the National Institute on Aging.

Age	Target Heart Rate
	(beats per minute)
40	126 - 153
50	119 - 145
60	112 - 136
70	105 - 128
80	98 - 119
90	91 - 111
100	84 – 102

Table 5.1. Target heart rates during aerobic exercise for different age groups

You can use a heart rate meter to check your pulse, or you can do it manually, feeling for the pulse beat at the base of your wrist, just below the ball of the thumb, or over one of your carotid arteries, on either side of your trachea. Do not count the pulse for one full minute, for it will slow down during this time. Instead, count it for ten seconds as soon as you stop exercising and multiply this number by six.

Straining Maneuvers

For those who are not able to stand or do any other exercise, research has found that repeated straining maneuvers are very effective in increasing the responsiveness of blood-pressure sensors. Called Valsalva maneuvers, they have been used by Air Force pilots who fly high-performance aircraft to protect them from fainting during steep turns that generate extremely high G-forces. They essentially involve sitting in a chair, straining abdominal muscles, and exhaling deeply at the same time, holding the strain for three seconds, resting for two seconds, and repeating this cycle of strain and rest for five repetitions. Pause for five minutes and repeat the cycle of five repetitions as many times as you can, up to a maximum of ten times.

A well-done Valsalva maneuver can raise blood pressure by approximately 50 mm Hg. I liken this straining maneuver to the test for lung function you are given at the doctor's office, when you are asked to blow as hard as you can into a tube connected to a measuring machine. Once mastered, it is very useful any time you stand up and begin to feel faint. It is not recommended for people with high blood pressure.

Lessons from Space

Who would have thought that something as simple as standing up, something we do spontaneously, would play so profound a role in keeping the blood-pressure control system primed—and that we would have discovered its importance by going into space?

In 1964, John Glenn used to jog five miles every day. He stopped jogging many years ago to avoid injury to his knees and hips. These days he stays fit with power walking—not race walking, but regular walking at a fast pace, swinging his arms vigorously. The emphasis here is on "regular" and "fast pace." Glenn power walks two miles daily, five days a week, and does upper-body weight training with dumbbells—"flies" (holding the weights in front of you, shoulder height, and opening your arms wide with elbows slightly bent) and biceps curls—for thirty minutes every other day. He emphasizes doing them slowly and correctly, exhaling deeply as you lift the weight.

If you watch John Glenn go about his business today, at eighty-three, you will notice that he does not spend much time sitting around.

6

Rhythms and Blues

Perfection in a clock does not consist in being fast but in being on time.

—*Marquis de Vauvenargues (1715–1747), Refléxions*

The cycles of day and night are the result of Earth's rotation as it orbits around the Sun. We see the Sun rise, set, and rise again every twenty-four hours. We measure our age by the number of these cycles from the day we were born. In all life on Earth there has evolved a genetic timing mechanism that reflects these cycles. Every cell in the body is attuned to this twenty-four-hour cycle of light and darkness and follows what is known as a "circadian rhythm," from the Latin words *circa* (about) and *dies* (a day). In humans, a pacemaker in the brain, activated by the length and intensity of daylight, synchronizes the body's responses. This sets up a daily pattern of changes in body temperature, heart rate, metabolic balance, and other functions, including the all-important cycle of sleeping and wakefulness.

But things are very different in space. As a spacecraft orbits Earth at an altitude greater than 100 miles (161 km), the cycle of daylight and darkness lasts only ninety minutes instead of twenty-four hours. The brain's biological clock cannot interpret this signal, because such an extremely short period is well outside the synchronizing range of humans—and indeed all other forms of life on Earth. The body's clock gets very confused. The timing of bodily functions goes its own way and they have a hard time working together. When it comes to organizing their work schedule, taking meals, or trying to get some sleep, astronauts try to ignore these frequent ninety minute day/nights. They stay on Houston time. Lights switch on and off inside the spacecraft, and their work and rest routines are regulated to give them roughly sixteen hours of lights-on and eight hours of lights-off.

But the trouble does not end there. Their body rhythms still drift, even when the shades are drawn. This implies that without gravity, light cues are not effective. Not infrequently, astronauts take some form of sleeping pill to help them sleep while they are in space. On the eighty-four-day *Skylab-4* mission, in 1973, Jerry Carr, Bill Pogue, and Ed Gibson took as many as four different kinds of sleep medication between them, including chloral hydrate, the chemical that was once secretly slipped into a drink called the "Mickey Finn" to render an unwitting subject unconscious. The fact that they tried so many kinds of sleep medication tells us just how difficult it was for these astronauts to get a good night's sleep.

How the System Works

In normal life on Earth, cues in the environment serve to synchronize the internal clock and to regulate the relationship of one body rhythm to another. This is not unlike what happens in an orchestra, where the individual musicians can all perform their own parts of the score but where the sound intended by the composer emerges only when they are all following the conductor's baton. So it is with body systems: to work properly, they must work in harmony.

The Rhythm of Life

Light is generally thought of as the strongest synchronizing cue on Earth—both its duration and intensity. Other cues that help to keep the biological clock in order are the daily habits that comprise our lives. Consistent times for waking and going to bed, set mealtimes, and the structured timetables of the workplace are strong reinforcing cues. So is spending time with individuals who have strongly synchronized rhythms—if you are older, spending more time with the young can be a powerful cue. And such cues are needed, because if they are not there, the biological clock can be thrown out of gear.

The Body's Clock

Even when the level of light is kept constant—by the imposition of continuous light or continuous darkness—and when an individual is isolated from other cues to the passing of time, the circadian rhythm of body functions persists, though the period becomes longer than twenty-four hours. This suggests that the body has its own internal biological clock. Although the rhythms of individual systems persist in such an isolated, time-free environment, they "free run"—that is, they lose their relationship to one another. The result is a whole gamut of health problems, including sleep disturbances, depression, eating disorders, susceptibility to colds and infections, loss of memory, and general confusion.

Is It Light or Is It Gravity?

The role of gravity is subtler. But experiencing the maximum pull of gravity, by alternating periods of activity and inactivity, can reinforce light and darkness' effect in synchronizing the various body rhythms. In fact, some scientists have long maintained that gravity rather than light may be the primary force that regulates circadian rhythms. They came to this view long before spaceflight was possible, by watching how the activity of small seashore crabs changes with the tides. The twice-daily rise and fall of the tides in the world's seas and oceans is produced by the gravitational attraction of the Moon and the Sun.

In space, where such gravity changes are absent but the internal light environment of the spacecraft is fairly normal, Tim Monk and his group at the University of Pittsburgh measured the rhythms in oral body temperature and alertness of astronaut Jerry Linenger on Space Station *Mir*. His internal clock seemed to function quite well throughout his first ninety days in space. Thereafter (days 110–120), his rhythms of body temperature and alertness were considerably weaker, with consequent disruptions in sleep. In my view, it is more likely that gravity and light cycles work together to reinforce the signal needed to synchronize body rhythms.

The Hormone That Sends You off to Dreamland

There is a very good reason for ensuring that day is as bright and night as dark as possible. Darkness stimulates the pineal gland in the brain to secrete the hormone melatonin, which helps you sleep. Light, by contrast, inhibits the production of melatonin and keeps you awake. Descartes, the seventeenth-century French philosopher, believed the pineal was the seat of the soul. Though this theory has been difficult to substantiate, the more recent discovery of the role of melatonin in inducing sleep has re-emphasized the importance of the pineal to physiology.

In the morning, an adequate degree of light intensity is necessary to inhibit melatonin production and kick-start the circadian day. This intensity should be over 2000 lux. (A lux is the standard international unit of illumination, taking into account both the intensity of a source of light and its distance from the user.) A typical well-lit office provides about 500 lux or less, but when outdoors on a sunny day people are exposed to more than 2000 lux over about four hours. An ordinary room would need quite a few 100-watt bulbs to provide the required intensity of light. I suppose one 100-watt bulb could probably approach 2000 lux if it were next to your nose. Regular light bulbs do not provide the wavelengths of sunlight, but lights that do so are commercially available.

The Rhythm of Sleep

Cycles of sleep and wakefulness are the most obvious of our daily rhythms. Sleep is the way the brain restores itself. It has had a hard day's work keeping all the body's systems and functions—temperature, breathing, heart rate, hormones, physical activity, and metabolism—at their peak. At the end of the day it needs to recharge itself and prepare for the next day's events. The functions it has been controlling reach their lowest point during the evening and night hours.

The kidneys slow down so that the need to urinate is suppressed during the night. In this way, Mother Nature allows an uninterrupted good night's rest. Thomas Dekker, the early seventeenth-century English dramatist, rightly observed that "sleep is the golden chain that ties health and our bodies together."

Paradoxically, sleep is the time when, in contrast to the body, the brain's electrical activity is highest. Sleep research pioneer Bill Dement, of Stanford University, proved that sleeping was "not just a human body in the 'off' position." Cycles of REM sleep (Rapid Eye Movement sleep, during which we dream) and non-REM sleep follow each other in a repeating pattern. Dement believed that "dreaming permits each and every one of us to be quietly and safely insane every night of our lives."

Each cycle of REM and non-REM sleep normally lasts about ninety minutes, during which there are five phases of distinct brainwave electrical activity. One of these, deep sleep (also known as slow-wave sleep), is the time when the body secretes growth hormone and does most of its healing and recovery.

The phase when we dream comes at the tail end of each REM sleep cycle and gets progressively longer during the night. It accounts for 10–25% of total sleep time. If we are not awakened between cycles by a full bladder, cold, worry, a loud noise, or some other disturbance, or by the dawn, we go into another ninety-minute cycle. A good balance between the five phases of sleep and the number of complete cycles is important to feeling refreshed when you wake up. Waking up, or being awakened, before a cycle is completed can leave you feeling exhausted.

How Much Sleep Do You Need?

There are no hard and fast rules concerning how much sleep we need. It was once believed that older people needed less sleep. However, Dement also showed that most people, whatever their age, need seven to eight hours a night, with women needing one hour more than men. There are always exceptions. Some people seem to be perfectly healthy with five hours' sleep, while others can sleep for ten hours without this indicating a health problem. Winston Churchill and Napoleon Bonaparte apparently needed only four hours, though Churchill was well known to be able to cat-nap at any spare moment of the day—during a train journey or a taxi ride or, in his later years, even during a parliamentary debate if the speakers bored him.

Have You Had a Good Night's Sleep?

Quality of sleep can be assessed in two ways. There is the subjective perception of feeling refreshed after a night's sleep and there is the objective measurement of brain waves during the sleep cycle. Whichever form of measurement is used, a good night's sleep begins with a short period of sleep latency—the time it takes to fall asleep. Some fall asleep the moment their head hits the pillow, but the count-down should be no more than twenty to thirty minutes from the time you are in bed and turn lights out. Those who consistently take longer than thirty minutes to fall asleep have a problem and need to see a doctor. A heavy meal late at night, leaving you with a very full stomach, can extend sleep latency, as can stress and a variety of other factors.

What Can Go Wrong?

Leaving on a Jet Plane

Working night shifts disturbs the harmony of body rhythms, and it takes several days of disturbed sleep, fatigue, confusion, slowed reflexes, and a general feeling of unease for these rhythms to readjust to the new sleep-work cycle. Those who alternate a few days of night shift with day shift never adjust and perpetually feel out of sorts.

Air travelers going rapidly through a number of time zones can similarly find, on landing, that their circadian rhythms have gone haywire. The condition is known as jet lag and recovery normally takes a few days.

What Can You do about Jet Lag

The more time zones you cross, the more days it takes to recover. It usually takes one day for each time zone (one hour) crossed. The amount of sleep you get during the flight determines how rested you will be when you arrive and how well you will adjust to the new environment.

It is tempting to drink alcohol on a plane, especially when it is served free of charge, as it is in first class, business class, and some long-haul economy flights. But alcohol has the effect of dehydrating the body, and jet lag is made much worse by dehydration. The humidity level in the cabin is very low once the plane is in the air, so dehydration is enough of a problem without being aggravated by alcohol. Avoid drinking altogether if you can, or restrict it to one small glass of red wine or cocktail and drink it early enough so that it is metabolized before you try to sleep. Coffee, too, is dehydrating and it keeps you awake. Drink lots of water or decaffeinated coffee instead.

The quality of sleep in a sitting position is not good. Most airplane cabins are darkened and quiet for only two or three hours, making a long stretch of sleep impossible. However, eye masks and earplugs are available for those who need them. If there are enough seats to stretch out, lie down to sleep. Even when sitting, cover your eyes and nap as much as you can. It is more difficult to sleep on a full stomach while a late dinner high in protein sits in your stomach longer. Eat a light dinner with little or no protein.

On boarding the plane, change your watch to the time of your destination so that you can adjust your mind to the new circadian phase. On arrival, carrying on as if you were still in the time frame of your point of origin hinders your body clock from resetting itself to the new location. Do as the locals do. If it's morning on arrival, take a shower to start off the day. Even better, a really hard exercise workout will do wonders in resetting your clock to the local time. If you are not up to that, however sleepy you feel, take a stroll in the park. A short siesta could be refreshing, but make sure it is no longer than ninety minutes. If you are attending a conference or a business meeting and tiredness starts to overwhelm you, stand or move about, and try to participate actively in the discussions.

Before going to bed, take a bath that is warm, but not hot. Take two aspirins or Ibuprofen (trade name Advil or Motrin) to help reduce your body temperature, which is at its lowest back home when you are asleep. Keep the lights dim before enjoying what now has a fair chance of being a sound night's sleep.

As we age, just as in space, the intensity of circadian cues may be diminished, either because we spend more time indoors with the curtains drawn or because we become less sensitive to them. As a result, we feel as if we were suffering from a kind of permanent low-level jet lag. We may be taking medications that fix one set of symptoms but throwing our body rhythms out of kilter in the process. It is not too surprising that older people sometimes become the victims of *polypharmacy*. This is the practice of taking handfuls of prescribed medications to treat an ever-increasing number of individual complaints, even though they probably all have a common underlying cause. Whatever the problem, it is likely to be helped by proper sleep.

Cumulative Sleep Loss

David Dinges at the University of Pittsburgh has found that as little as twenty minutes less sleep per day than the seven or eight hours considered normal will result in a cumulative sleep loss that affects performance over a period of several days. Sleep deprivation is estimated to cause one in four traffic accidents. Analyses of the *Challenger* Shuttle accident in 1986 and the Chernobyl nuclear power plant explosion that same year have revealed that sleep deprivation and exhaustion of the workforce were contributing factors.

What Keeps You Awake?

Some 40 million Americans suffer from chronic sleep problems. Two of the more extreme are narcolepsy, characterized by sudden, uncontrollable sleepiness, and its opposite, severe insomnia, due to depression or nightmares that cause sleepers to wake up worried and anxious. More common, however, are complaints from older people that they are sleeping less during the night, with increased dozing off during the day. In addition, the little sleep they do get is often shallow and fragmented by long waking episodes. These reduce the stages of deep sleep and alter the distribution of REM sleep throughout the night.

Spontaneous waking has many causes. It could arise from the need to urinate or it could be associated with sleep apnea, a condition in which people wake up during the night because they have stopped breathing. This is due to slack neck muscles obstructing their air passages. Apnea could also be the result of drinking a little too much alcohol before going to bed or taking medication for asthma or a cold, some of which are full of stimulants that keep would-be sleepers awake. In women who are passing through the menopause, it could be related to hot flashes.

Caffeine, a powerful stimulant, finds its way into many foods and drinks. Yes, everyone knows someone who has no problem falling asleep after drinking coffee, but it keeps most of us awake. A cup of coffee contains a powerful sleep-busting charge of 110 mg caffeine, a small bowl of coffee ice cream contains 58 mg, and an 8 oz can of Coca-Cola contains 23 mg. Though many people are careful about drinking decaffeinated coffee in the evening, they may not be aware that they are getting a substantial shot of caffeine if they choose coffee ice cream. Cocoa and chocolate contain theobromine, a relative of caffeine. It is also a stimulant, though it is weaker than caffeine.

Sleep in Space

Upset rhythms lead to disturbed sleep. Disturbed sleep is a common complaint aboard all spacecraft. This is not helped by the heavy workload. It takes longer to do things in space and there is so much to do that astronauts work very long days—often more than sixteen hours. In 1965, the *Gemini VII* crewmen reported feeling fatigued. They slept an average of only 5.3 hours a night, and sleep was particularly poor on the first night, a fact reported by numerous astronauts. During the last four days, they slept less than five hours a night. In general, Shuttle astronauts are known to sleep one to three hours less a night in space than they would on Earth.

In addition to the telescoped day/night cycle, there are many conditions aboard all spacecraft that are not conducive to a good night's sleep. The noise level from fans and motors is high. Even when asleep, astronauts remain particularly sensitive to changes in this noise level, especially if it stops! This is not unlike new parents being sensitive to their baby's sounds at night.

The astronauts' unusual schedules may decrease sleep duration, displace the time when sleep occurs, and interfere with its quality. But overall, the most significant changes in sleep occur not in flight but upon return to Earth's gravity. The alterations are more in the quality of their sleep than in its quantity.

On *Neurolab*, the 1998 Shuttle research mission dedicated to the Decade of the Brain, Chuck Czeisler at Harvard University Medical School monitored sleep from the ground on three nights during the sixteen-day mission. He was surprised to find that astronauts slept a full eight hours and that their sleep was remarkably normal, whereas on the nights when Czeisler did not monitor sleep, the activity meters worn by astronauts indicated that they got only five to six hours' sleep. It appears that when they were not being monitored, they allowed their activities in space to encroach upon the time allocated for sleeping.

Living quarters aboard a spacecraft are very tight, but astronauts are now provided with individual sleep bunkers. These bunkers are now quieter than other parts of the ship and have provided an adequate period of darkness, uninterrupted by the ninety-minute sunrise and sunset with each orbit.

Astronauts comment that although they generally sleep well in terms of duration, they do not feel rested when they wake up. On nights when they sleep poorly, this affects them even more the next day than comparable sleep loss on Earth would. Oleg Atkov, a Russian cardiovascular specialist who flew on *Salyut 7* for 236 days in 1984, complained that difficulty sleeping was the worst part of his space experience. When probed further, he commented that "in space, you could not feel like you put your head down on a pillow, as you do on Earth, and even if you had slept many hours, you did not feel refreshed when you woke up."

What Part Does Gravity Play in Sleep?

The part that gravity plays in sleeping deserves a fuller consideration. We do not know why putting our heads down contributes to a good night's sleep. Yet we do know that except for the occasional nap, we get much more refreshing sleep that way than if we fall asleep in a chair or standing up which is next to impossible unless you are extremely tired. When we stand or when we sit, the weight of the head is supported atop the rest of the body. Blood is pulled away from the head and the body has to work harder to get it back to the head. When we lie down, gravity is pulling directly on the head instead of the feet. Blood shifts towards the head.

Lying down also reduces the activity of the sympathetic nervous system. In fact, its counterpart, the parasympathetic nervous system, led by the powerful vagus nerve, takes over, slowing the heartbeat and breathing. The demands on the body are reduced and the brain is able to recharge itself during sleep.

At the Ends of the Earth

In Polar regions, where the days are extremely long in the summer and very, very short in the winter, sleep difficulties are a common problem. In northern Scandinavian countries and in northern Alaska and Canada, increased depression, suicides, and crime are not uncommon during the dark winter months.

The early Antarctic exploring parties noted that although the total daily quantity of sleep did not differ, its quality and pattern did, and the occurrence of insomnia at night increased. This has been confirmed in recent years in personnel stationed for months in Arctic and Antarctic outposts. Their sleep quality deteriorated so much that only the lightest stages of sleep were ever reached. Deep sleep practically disappeared, and the dream phase of sleep was significantly reduced. Those who were deprived of a fully satisfying night's sleep reported that they felt withdrawn, easily annoyed, and preoccupied with vague physical discomforts. They also suffered from varying degrees of depression.

Having to Get Up in the Middle of the Night

As can happen in old age, astronauts in space and volunteers in bed-rest find that the urge to urinate comes on strongly in the middle of the night. Physician astronaut Drew Gaffney told me he could not enjoy a good night's sleep when he got back from his Shuttle flight of seven days in 1991 because of this need (whose medical name is *nocturnal diuresis*). It took him four to six days to recover completely.

The wife of another astronaut told me that on his first night back home after he had flown for only five days on the Shuttle, she was awakened by a thump. Her husband had fallen to the floor when he tried to *float* to the bathroom, as he had done in space. For a young man in his thirties, the need to urinate in the night is most unusual. It is not known whether other astronauts have had similar experiences, since they go home soon after landing and do not think it significant enough to report.

What Disturbs Sleep?

With advancing age we often see earlier bedtimes and earlier awakenings. Some scientists say this is probably due to a shortening of the twenty-four-hour period of one's internal biological clock. However, those who have always been early risers, by choice or because of work routines, do not usually report such changes. It is not too surprising that many hard-working people who look forward to sleeping in after retirement find they still wake up at 5 or 6 A.M. Whether they do so or not also depends on how structured their retired life turns out to be, how much time they spend outdoors, and how active they remain. One always sleeps better after an active day.

The tendency of older people to stay indoors may deprive their body clock of a natural reference point. At least two hours outside in the sunlight are needed to keep this clock in good working order. Scott Campbell at Cornell University, in New York, and Sonia Ancoli-Israel at the University of California, in San Diego, found that in general, elderly men living at home were exposed to ninety minutes of sunlight per day, and women forty-five minutes. Patients with Alzheimer's living at home got just thirty minutes, and elderly patients in nursing homes often had as little as two minutes.

Sending the Body Rhythms Haywire

Continuous bed-rest is a form of sensory deprivation. It eliminates the regular daily alteration between activity and rest and reduces the number of variations in the pull of gravity on the body associated with constant changes of position—from lying to standing or sitting to standing, for instance. This is similar to what happens to older people when they cease to be active. The stability of circadian rhythms deteriorates in healthy young bed-rest volunteers even when the brain is provided with such other cues as regular mealtimes and regular changes between light and darkness. Body rhythms begin to lose their synchronization after as little as ten days in bed, and the disruption reaches its height after twenty-two to twenty-four days.

For example, it has been observed in bed-rest studies that the rhythm of the hormone insulin is inverted. Normally, it peaks during the day, keeping the level of blood sugar under control. During bed rest, insulin secretion peaks at night, which is not healthy—for among other things, it inhibits the normal secretion of human growth hormone during deep sleep. Eating a high-sugar meal shortly before going to bed has the same effect.

Regulating the Thermostat

One of the most basic causes of friction among couples is the temperature setting of the thermostat! Men prefer it cooler than women. The ability to respond to a temperature challenge can also be affected by one's level of fitness and age. Astronauts and older persons have trouble adjusting to sharp changes in temperature. In both cases, as in bed-rest, there is less increase in blood flow to the skin and less sweating to cool the skin down in response to heat. With reduced blood volume, less blood flow, and a lower ability to dissipate heat, astronauts, not unlike the elderly, feel cold even in 80° F temperatures.

Under normal conditions, body temperature is at its maximum in the afternoon, one hour later than the time of maximum heart rate in men but at the same time in women. Sleepiness is triggered by, among other factors, a drop in temperature late at night. But during long-term bed-rest, the time gap between the two peaks of heart rate and body temperature can increase by as much as eight hours, so body temperature is still relatively high at the time the bed-rest volunteers should be falling asleep.

To Nap or Not to Nap

The inability to sleep through the night may be the result of frequent napping during the day. But it is hard to say which is cause and which is effect. John Glenn certainly had no time to nap while he was training for his *STS-95* flight in 1998 and at the same time fulfilling all his senatorial duties. Before his flight, he had to spend a night in Chuck Czeisler's sleep lab in Boston. Glenn amazed everybody by sleeping a full eight hours. Commenting on his results, Czeisler said, "Prior to the mission, [Glenn's] sleep assessment was appropriate for a normal healthy individual without sleep complaints. Throughout the mission, however…he showed less sleep time and increased wakefulness." This is not an unusual pattern during spaceflight.

Do You Stop Breathing while You Sleep?

There is a link between sleep and respiration. Sleep apnea (brief interruptions of breathing during sleep) is a serious, potentially life-threatening condition that becomes increasingly likely with age. Its symptoms include snoring, choking sensations due to cessation of breathing, and waking up repeatedly. All this leads to excessive daytime sleepiness. It is believed that most victims of sleep apnea remain undiagnosed and untreated. There may be as many as twelve to fifteen million in the U.S. alone.

It was predicted that astronauts would suffer sleep apnea in space. The shift of abdominal contents upward, because of the absence of gravity, would affect respiration by increasing the obstruction of air passages. This would lead to disturbed sleep. Surprisingly, this has not happened. In fact, fewer episodes of apnea than expected were recorded in space even though snoring has occasionally been heard against the background noise of the fans and motors!

Healthy young men in continuous bed-rest begin to complain of sleep problems within two or three days. They recall colorful, vivid dreams that they normally did not experience, or at least did not remember, before the bed-rest began. They take longer to fall asleep and wake frequently during the night. When they awaken in the morning, they report feelings of fatigue, irritability, and confusion and find it hard to concentrate. Grumpy old men and ill-tempered old women could well be victims of poor sleeping.

Getting the Blues

Older people who do not go out much and live sedentary lives in subdued lighting are prime candidates for depression, which often goes hand in hand with sleep problems. The assumption of many doctors, senior caregivers, and family members is that depression is an inevitable part of growing older. After all, many elderly people see themselves gradually going downhill. They may feel worthless physically and mentally, and attempts to talk them out of that belief may have proven futile. Robert Butler, the first director of the National Institute on Aging and now the head of The International Longevity Center, a New York think tank on aging issues, says, "The worst pieces of advice an older person can receive are 'What do you expect at your age?' and 'Take it easy.'"

At some time or another we all know what it is to have the blues. Sometimes we know the reason—being dumped by a loved one, being fired from a job, or just being broke. We usually get over it and set about picking up the pieces of our lives. At other times, we feel sad or anxious and cry for no apparent reason. Again, the passage of time usually heals this melancholy condition. While it lasts, depression is a mental illness that affects mood, sleep patterns, thought, behavior, and energy levels.

Our forefathers had doubt that gravity, especially the Moon's gravity, could affect a person's mental state. The word "lunatic," which is no longer in technical use, comes from the Latin *lunaticus,* meaning moonstruck. The relationship of gravity to depression is most likely the result of the pronounced inactivity that is associated with this disorder. But contrary to popular belief, depression is treatable whatever its severity.

The Curse of Depression

Clinical depression is usually seen in people with a family history of mood disorders. Its victims cannot cope with situations and events that others would take in stride. This is the most severe type of depression. It can go on for months or even years, and if left untreated it can lead to suicide. Working on a project in the early 1970s with a group of depressive patients at the Palo Alto Veterans Hospital in Palo Alto, California, I got a first-hand view of the disease. A patient sitting in her chair was given a comb and asked to comb her hair. The emotional struggle she went through trying to raise that comb to her head—without success—made an impression I will never forget.

A human being in the grip of depression feels empty, hopeless, worthless, lonely, and desperate. Ordinary activities bring no pleasure. Sleep does not come easily. Depressed people stand out at a distance, because they neglect their appearance. They have difficulty concentrating, remembering, and making decisions, and they seem to live perpetually on the gloomy side of the street.

At Christmas, and other festive times, things only get worse. Surrounded by family and friends who are laughing, singing, and enjoying one another's company only deepens the inner sadness that depressed people are already experiencing. What they are going through is not unlike a period of grieving. Many withdraw for three or four days to the solitude of a room with curtains drawn, staring at TV for hours on end. Some now go to churches that offer long Blue Christmas services as a refuge. The suicide rate is particularly high during such holidays.

Seasonal depression is a much milder form that particularly affects people during the winter months, when days are short and there is not much sunshine. This type of depression is common in areas such as Seattle, where there are relatively few hours of sunlight and little respite from long periods of dull, cloudy, wet weather. It is also seen in regions such as Alaska or the Scandinavian countries, which are within or close to the Arctic Circle. The days are extremely short in the winter, and sometimes people live in continuous night for the better part of six months. The suicide rate peaks at these times in these countries. Bright-light treatment, which can reset the biological clock, has been clinically useful for people who suffer from seasonal depression.

There are 17 million diagnosed depressed persons in the USA, yet there are many who are not diagnosed and do not receive treatment. By no means are all of them elderly, but as many as 3% of the nation's sixty-five-year-olds may be considered clinically depressed, while many more suffer from seasonal depression. The common wisdom is that depression is a one-way street in the elderly. However, mild depression is very treatable.

Why Do We Get Depressed?

There is little point in admonishing a truly depressed person by saying, "For goodness' sake, snap out of it and cheer up!" for the condition is directly linked to chemical changes in the brain. The messenger chemicals serotonin and norepinephrine, which normally carry instructions from neuron to neuron, are out of balance, so the ability of the brain's circuits to convey messages breaks down. These changes show up in brain scans. Magnetic Resonance Imaging (MRI) reveals shrinkage in the prefrontal cortex of depressives and other people with mood disorders. No one knows whether this shrinkage is the cause of the disease or its result. Scans have also shown that blood flow through the brain is reduced in depressives, and this finding has been used as a marker, or indication, of the disease.

In Space, Excitement Can Banish Depression

Depression has not been identified as a problem in spaceflight. Certainly, on short flights there is little time to become depressed. There is too much excitement about achieving one's lifetime goals, and there is the simple thrill of being in space. The crew will have trained together for at least a year and become a very tightly knit group. The experiments and other work that must be accomplished in the highly unusual environment of minimal gravity, where nothing stays put, gives them more than enough to do and leaves no time to brood.

On flights of longer duration, such as those on Russia's *Mir* or on the International Space Station, there is more time for introspection and therefore greater potential for depression. Astronauts separated from their loved ones on Earth, and perhaps emotionally or culturally isolated from their crewmates, can get the feeling that the world, and even ground control, have forgotten them.

Shannon Lucid, the U.S. astronaut who in 1996 spent 120 days on the Russian spacecraft *Mir*, was prepared for the experience. She equipped herself with reading material, exercised regularly, and developed excellent team spirit with her male Russian crewmates. Shannon used e-mail to stay in touch with family and friends. And when she felt she did not have enough to do, she asked for more experiments to be sent up.

Others have fared less well, losing more weight than is normal and experiencing withdrawal and loneliness. They felt picked on, abandoned by those on the ground, irritable, and in conflict with their fellow astronauts. Some quietly left NASA after returning. Others were more vocal and have even written books and magazine articles about their disappointments. Cosmonaut Oleg Atkov, who was up there for six months, has described how his feelings towards his crewmates in 1984 alternated between the closest camaraderie and hostility. But the crew was drawn together by their hostility towards the cosmonaut who brought up mail and supplies, since he was going back home to Earth after only a few days while they were stuck in space.

On Earth, Inactivity Can Deepen Gloom

A period of bed-rest as short as two to four weeks can produce similar feelings of isolation. In the late 1960s, when I was carrying out bed-rest studies in preparation for the Skylab missions, I was amazed by the dramatic change in the attitudes and moods of the male volunteers. These studies involved fifty-six days of continuous bed rest, and when the volunteers first came in they all had ambitious plans. They were going to read the books they had never gotten around to reading before, learn a foreign language, and take a college course for credit.

By the twentieth day they had gone strangely quiet. They were no longer interested in their surroundings or their appearance, in the activities and chatter of staff or visitors, in hearing news of the outside world, or in reading or even in receiving mail. Their sense of time was distorted. When it was time to have blood drawn, or to eat lunch, they just lay there, awake but unemotional. A few had to be fed. It was an effort for them to engage in conversation.

These symptoms disappeared when they got out of bed. Once they resumed using gravity to the full they gradually regained their good spirits, and they were back to normal by the time they went home twenty days later. Russian scientists carrying out bed-rest studies that lasted 62 and 120 days made similar observations.

Such symptoms seem to crop up wherever human beings have undergone long periods of isolation or confinement. Teams wintering over in Antarctic stations, the crews of nuclear submarines, and workers on Norwegian oil rigs in the North Sea have all shown signs of withdrawal. In all these cases, however, as the time to return to normal life approaches, there is a renewed interest in appearance, personal hygiene, and exercise.

The Mid-Life Crisis

The conditions that cause the symptoms of depression in all these cases are not too dissimilar to the changes in lifestyle that come with advancing years. The symptoms may show up as early as the menopause in women. They can affect men in their fifties as well. When they are reinforced by feelings that one's body is deteriorating and that one's worth in the workplace is diminishing, this state has come to be known as the male mid-life crisis.

It is all too easy for an older person to become inactive, to spend more and more time in bed or sitting in a chair in subdued light, to avoid or forget to go outdoors, and to end up feeling abandoned by family and friends. Attending funerals can become the most common social function. But there is no need to accept a lifestyle that invites depression.

The factors contributing to depression among the elderly include poor health, medications taken to reduce blood pressure, low self-esteem, the loss of a partner, money problems, and moving out of a much-loved home. The biggest obstacles to recovery are a negative attitude and the feeling of being too old or too unworthy to seek help.

If every morning the first page you turn to in the newspaper is the one that carries the obituaries, to see which contemporary has abandoned you today, it is probably time to take stock and change your ways. If you have given up the effort to harness gravity by remaining active, you enter a vicious cycle that has only one end—unless you break out of it. Being active has proven very beneficial in combating depression. The sooner even a mild depression is identified, the more effectively the progression to severe depression will be forestalled.

What Can You Do about It?

It is not unusual for elderly people to doze off throughout the day. If they fall asleep without turning the lights out, their circadian rhythms will drift or free run, and sleep will be disturbed because the lights will be keeping their melatonin down.

Such habits are not restricted to the elderly—they are not uncommon among college students, though for different reasons. A student may have been at a party the night before, or may have stayed up all night studying for a test. Bad sleeping habits affect health by suppressing the immune system and increasing sensitivity to infections. Both college students and the elderly are more prone to infections than the general population. But anybody suffering the effects of disturbed sleep can probably be helped. Sleep that leaves you feeling refreshed restores your energy and can make you look better and live longer.

Things to Do—and to Avoid—as Bedtime Draws Near

Exercise earlier in the day rather than later at night. This gives your body temperature time to come down and so helps you to sleep. Sexual activity is an exception to the rule about exercise. It is great sleep therapy probably because it is followed by total relaxation.

Do not eat or drink anything containing caffeine after mid-afternoon. This includes coffee, caffeinated soft drinks, iced tea, coffee ice cream, and caffeine-containing remedies for colds and headaches, such as Dristan or Excedrin. Nicotine is a stimulant too, so try not to smoke.

Do not eat a heavy meal late at night, especially one containing lots of protein.

Tried and trusted bedtime relaxation techniques such as taking a warm bath, drinking hot milk, and listening to quiet music can work wonders. Milk, especially buttermilk, is rich in tryptophan, the amino acid parent of serotonin, the brain's chemical transmitter responsible for sleep.

To reduce the need to empty your bladder during the night, limit what you drink for the last two hours before going to bed. Especially avoid drinking too much alcohol. You may fall asleep faster, but after an hour or two you are likely to wake up—and stay awake.

Do not bring your worries to bed. Build a mental wall between daytime activities and night by planning your next day and talking through any problems long before you go to bed. Do not allow anyone to upset you or ask you to solve a problem for two hours before going to bed. Set aside some time in the early afternoon to do your worrying if you have to, but try not to worry if there is nothing you can do about the problem.

• Make a Ritual of Bedtime

Go to bed and get up at the same time every day. Your body will develop its own sleep rhythms. Remember that you have gone to bed to relax and to sleep—not to watch TV. Meditate, sit quietly, and imagine yourself in a relaxing place. This helps your brainwave patterns to mimic the early stages of sleep.

Do not fall asleep with the lights on. Sleep in bed, not in a chair. If you read in bed, aim the reading light at the book, not at your face, and keep the light intensity as low as you can manage without straining your eyes. Choose reading material that does not make you anxious or irritated.

Open a window as weather permits. If you are awakened in the middle of the night by a full bladder, turning on a bright bathroom light could cause you to spend the next two hours wide awake, fretting that you cannot fall asleep. Use the bathroom nightlight.

If you wake up too early and want to try to go back to sleep, say some repetitive prayer to yourself—or a poem if you are not a believer. Counting sheep never worked for me.

• Regulating the Light Environment

Research in humans and other primates has shown that ideally there should be sixteen hours of light to eight hours darkness to synchronize circadian rhythms. Get plenty of light during the day and ensure that night is as dark as possible. During the day, take care that there is always plenty of bright light indoors, either from the sun or from artificial lighting. Try to spend a fair amount of your time outdoors. If your room has lots of natural light, get blackout shades or curtains for the night.

Do not sit in bright light for the two hours before going to bed. Instead, sit in dimmed or indirect light. Do not turn bright lights on in the bathroom. Bathroom lights are usually brighter than those in other rooms of a home, so a dimmer switch or a nightlight is a good idea.

• Bright Light Treatment

Astronauts have used exposure to bright lights (2,500–10,000 lux) before they go into space as a means of shifting their circadian rhythms closer to the new light/dark schedules they will be entering. Such bright-light treatment has proved effective in helping resynchronize rhythms and so helping people to sleep. It has also proven useful in treating some types of depression.

Elderly people, especially those living in some form of community housing, often get little or no bright light during the day. At night, they are surrounded by increased activity and noise and may well be exposed to ambient light, as lights in rooms and hallways are switched on by staff. As a result, they experience problems with their circadian rhythms and suffer from disturbed sleep. People in this age group may already be taking many medications, and sleeping pills are often of little or no value to them.

Bright-light therapy consists of sitting for thirty minutes to two hours while reading or engaged in some other activity, in front of a box of special lights. The box looks much like a computer screen, containing a bank of high-intensity white fluorescent light bulbs that mimic the wavelength characteristics of sunlight, but without the ultraviolet radiation, and provide up to 10,000 lux. This is three or four times the maximum light intensity that one would normally get on a bright summer's day and far beyond what could be achieved with 100-watt bulbs.

Improvement has been reported within two weeks of treatment. Depending on individual needs, as little as 4,000–5,000 lux may suffice after the initial treatment. Research studies beyond four weeks have not been done. Light boxes for home use are available commercially by mail or through the internet, from sources such as the Environmental Medicine Company, in Vancouver, Canada (trade name Bio-Light Boxes), or The Sunbox Company in Gaithersburg, Maryland (trade name Sun-A-Lux Box).

• Cat-napping

Catnapping is not a bad thing if it is structured into your daily routine; but it should not be random. It should be restricted to fifteen to ninety minutes and should not be too close to normal bed time. Sara Medwick at Harvard University, in Boston, says the brain may require the time out that a nap provides. Even in young people doing repetitive tasks like typing, she found that performance deteriorated after several hours but was restored by an hour's nap. My copy editor reports that an afternoon nap is highly beneficial in his profession as well which requires intense concentration. An afternoon siesta is a well-established practice in many Latin and Mediterranean countries, such as Greece, Italy, and Spain. It is regarded there as a healthy, refreshing habit.

• The Snoring Problem

If you snore, believe you suffer from sleep apnea (episodes of breathlessness during sleep), or tend to doze off during the day or while driving, make sure you get the problem diagnosed properly. Taking sleeping pills could be dangerous. Changing your sleeping position, losing weight, or abstaining from alcohol may help. In extreme conditions, surgery has been used. Most people find relief and a good night's rest for themselves and their partner by wearing a special mask over the nose during sleep. The mask is attached to a supply of pressurized air via a blower that forces the air through the nasal passages.

• Melatonin Supplements

Supplements of melatonin have been promoted as the cure-all sleep medication. They can be bought without a prescription at health-food stores. Some people claim melatonin is also an anti-aging remedy and an antioxidant. Neither of these claims has been proven. Melatonin supplements may help some people to sleep if their insomnia is caused by disturbed rhythms, as with jet lag, but not if it is due to anxiety, apnea, or other causes. If it is taken at the wrong time, it can disrupt the sleeping/waking cycle. The dose that is effective in inducing sleep is a fraction of the 3 mg tablets sold at stores, which can send blood levels of melatonin soaring to forty times higher than normal. In this case, more is definitely not better. The side effects include confusion, drowsiness, and headache the next morning. Research suggests that melatonin may cause blood vessels to constrict—a dangerous consequence for anybody with high blood pressure. Regulating your light environment so as to allow your own body-produced melatonin to do its job is cheaper, more effective, and safer.

• Other Drugs

Drugs have their place in treating severe insomnia, but as a last resort and only for short periods of time. Sleeping medications such as the benzodiazepines (trade names Valium, Temazepan, Normison, Mogadon, Rohypnol) are addictive and are not recommended for long-term treatment. Herbs such as chamomile tea or valerian are safe alternatives.

• If All Else Fails...

If despite everything you still cannot sleep, get up and give yourself the satisfaction of getting ahead on your chores. Perhaps you can carry out some task that would otherwise have gone undone. I have found cleaning fits that category well. But remember to take a short nap after lunch—no more than ninety minutes.

Feeling Blue for No Apparent Reason

If you believe you are experiencing any of the symptoms of depression, see your doctor and get diagnosed properly. Never make the mistake of believing you are beyond cure. There are standard ways of treating this illness, and they are set out below.

• Talking to an Expert

Talking with a trained therapist, counselor, or psychotherapist is a good first step. In cases of very mild depression, it may be the only treatment needed. The National Institute of Mental Health (NIMH) recommends structured treatment of about twelve to twenty sessions of cognitive therapy and/or interpersonal therapy. The first of these methods involves acquiring knowledge and an understanding of the disease by reasoning, intuition, and perception. The second focuses on how you relate to other people. You are helped to recognize and change negative thinking patterns. Then the therapy shifts to helping you to improve relationships and interact more effectively with other people. Re-structuring one's life by revising priorities, modifying a way of thinking and behavior can go a long way in reducing depressive symptoms at any age.

• Drugs

The drugs most often used to treat depression in the past included imipramine (trade name Tofranil), phelzine (Nardil), and tranylcypromine (Parnate). Since then, a number of new drugs that are more effective and have fewer side effects have become available. Among them are fluoxetine (trade name Prozac), citalopram (Celexa), venlafaxine (Effexor), paroxetine (Paxil), and sartaline (Zoloft). They all act by allowing the brain's mood-controlling chemicals, norepinephrine, or the feel good substance, serotonin, to accumulate at nerve endings and so stimulate the brain cells. This results in improved mood, higher energy levels, increased ability to concentrate, a healthier appetite, and better patterns of sleep.

Some 60 to 70% of patients respond to the first antidepressant they take, but about 10 to 15% do not respond at all to these drugs. Sometimes more than one drug is needed. Many foods interact with the drugs taken for depression. Red wine, beer, cheese, salami or pepperoni, raisins, bananas, and avocados should be avoided, because in combination with the drugs they can increase blood pressure and cause dizziness or drowsiness.

It usually takes two to four weeks of drug treatment before someone who is depressed begins to feel better. If the drugs are discontinued this must be done gradually and no other antidepressant should be taken for at least two weeks. It is not known why it takes so long to see improvements. One explanation may be that it takes time to resynchronize the biological rhythms that are disturbed during depression—just as it takes time to recover from jet lag.

In Europe, the herb St. John's Wort has been used to treat depression. Is use has not yet been approved by the Food and Drug Administration (FDA) in the U.S., although it is readily available at health-food stores without a prescription. The National Institute of Mental Health (NIMH) is conducting a rigorous series of studies into the benefits and possible side effects of St. John's Wort, and it is trying to isolate its major chemical components to determine what is responsible for its effects on the brain.

• Short, Sharp Shocks

In earlier centuries, doctors believed that treatments aiming at *shaking up the system* would help mental patients "snap out of it." Medical science has advanced since then, and treatments have become more sophisticated, but the principle of the short, sharp shock has survived. In today's world, it is expected to re-synchronize brain and body rhythms.

Hypergravity This treatment was used in the nineteenth century, but its success rate cannot have been high, because it did not stand the test of time. Patients were spun around fast on a hand-cranked centrifuge in order to subject them to high gravity levels. Despite its falling out of fashion, with today's advances in technology and our better understanding of how the brain works, hypergravity warrants a second look.

Electric Shock Therapy Until antidepressant drugs were discovered and chlorpromazine was introduced in 1951, the only effective treatment against severe depression was to pass an electric current through the brain. Electroconvulsive Therapy (ECT) was crude and dangerous at first, but improved procedures have made this treatment much safer. It is used when rapid improvement is required, when depression is extremely severe, or when drugs do not work.

Bright Light Bright-light treatment, used to treat sleep problems, can also be effective against mild to moderate depression and seasonal depression. Daily exposure early in the morning, with the light intensity at 10,000 lux, has been found useful. Sessions lasting from half an hour to two hours should produce results after two weeks.

• Aerobic Exercise

Another old prescription that is receiving a resurgence of interest as a means of treating depression is regular aerobic exercise—that is, exercise hard enough to force you to be out of breath and to sweat. Depressed people usually have a reduced flow of blood to the brain, and brain scans show that aerobic exercise can restore the flow to normal. Think of it as a form of jogging for the brain—a way of repairing the neurochemical imbalance that can cause depression.

Exercise makes you feel good even if you are not depressed. However, a leisurely stroll in the park is not going to do the trick. Byrum Kerasu, who heads the Task Force on the Treatment of Depression for the American Psychiatric Association, in New York City, is a firm believer in the curative power of vigorous exercise. His recommendations range from sixteen minutes on a treadmill at 3 mph on a 4-degree uphill grade, working up to one hour.

Kerasu goes as far as to propose that exercise will one day replace psychotherapy and drugs as a cure for depression. There is solid evidence why that should be so. As long ago as the 1960s and 1970s, daily exercise was shown to increase the brain chemicals norepinephrine and serotonin in rats and norepinephrine in the blood of people aged sixty-five to sixty-nine. Exercise produced an increase in the number of blood vessels in the brain. In general, whereas small immediate effects were seen with all types of exercise, the largest impact on depression was found in exercise programs that lasted seventeen weeks or longer. What this really means is that to be effective, exercise—another word for harnessing gravity—must become a lifetime habit.

• Restructure Your Life

For mild depression, which is more likely to be encountered among elderly people than the severe form, making the effort to change your lifestyle is a far better option than taking drugs. Take a good look at the way you live, at the environment you live in, and at your level of activity. If something strikes you as being wrong, take immediate steps to remedy the situation. Establish consistent patterns for bedtimes and mealtimes. Spend as much time as possible outdoors. Let the sunlight into your home. To the best of your ability, spend sixteen hours in the light and eight hours in darkness. Join an exercise class, or at least become more active in your own home and garden.

A Footnote from Thomas Jefferson

The ancient Greeks set themselves the ideal of "a healthy mind in a healthy body." Thomas Jefferson, a great lover of classical Greece, adopted this advice when he wrote, "Not less than two hours a day should be devoted to exercise, and the weather little regarded. I speak this from experience, having made this arrangement of my life. If the body is feeble, the mind will not be strong."

7

Brain, Mind, and Memory

○ ○

The mind, of course, is just what the brain does for a living.

—*Sharon Begley, editor, Newsweek magazine*

Before cosmonaut Valery Polyakov was ready to make his trip to the Russian space station *Mir* in 1994 for his historic record breaking fourteen-month stay in space, he had to learn more than 5,000 English technical terms. Generally, his English was good. As a medical doctor, he often used it to read scientific papers and communicate with his colleagues in the West. But technical engineering terms were a different matter. He had worked long and hard to master these terms, which were after all critical to his survival on the spacecraft.

The launch went beautifully, the docking of the Soyuz to the *Mir*, perfect. But, as he tells the story, after a few days of living in space, he could not remember a single one of the 5,000 terms. He remembered his English, but the technical terms had gone. He tried all kinds of mental exercises to recall them but to no avail. One day, some six weeks after he had launched, they started to come back.

Questions That Need Answers

What happened to Valery Polyakov? Had this happened to others? Not many may be as candid as Polyakov. Maybe his loss of memory was brought on by the stress of his mission, for stress is known to cause temporary amnesia. Did gravity have anything to do with it? This would not be too surprising, though it is not a question that has been explored in any depth. In areas of mind and emotions, astronauts are not very forthcoming in sharing how they feel. Astronauts will have to be more open about their emotional experiences to help us address potential problems that will arise on a long trip to Mars..

141

Emotions have a very powerful effect on memory. We tend to remember more vividly those events we associate with a strong, pleasant emotional experience, such as falling in love. Conversely, anxiety, fear, and stress can impair memory. Some experiences can be so horrifying and distressing—being on a battlefield and under fire for days on end, for instance—that they are deleted from the memory, or sent to some destination from which they can be retrieved only with the help of a skilled therapist. Many times the fear of losing your memory in itself can interfere with the ability to remember, even though there is nothing wrong with your memory per se.

The Computer and the Pizza

It is becoming a cliché to describe the brain as the central computing unit of the body, but no computer yet built can match it. Researchers at the Massachusetts Institute of Technology (MIT), near Boston, and at the University of California, Berkeley, have been battling for the last thirty years over whether or not such a machine could even exist.

Rodney Brooks directs the 230-person MIT Artificial Intelligence Laboratory, which argues that a super-smart computer can be developed that can be just as complex, and just as fast, as the brain—and with the capability of doing every-thing the brain does. Hubert Dreyfus and John Searle at Berkeley have pointed out that though a computer might perform most of the brain's more mechanical functions, it would still not be conscious. The following is one of Seale's favorite analogies in describing such a computer: "A computer program simulating the brain would no more be able to be conscious than a computer simulating diges-tion would be able to actually eat a pizza."

The brain has many other attributes that seem to put it in a class of its own, far ahead of any challenger, at this stage at least. A computer can play chess, but could it ever fall in love? Display intuition? Show initiative (though sometimes I suspect mine does)? Apply common sense to a problem? Feel good or get the blues? Experience faith? Have such human feelings as pride, self-confidence, or shyness? Make a decision that defies logic?

The Dark Side of the Moon

This debate of whether a computer is as good as a human has carried through to space. The issue is whether to continue to send humans to explore space or to rely entirely on robots. The dimension of the human mind's contribution was dem-onstrated vividly during the 1969–1972 Apollo missions, when astronauts landed on the Moon six times, in six different locations. Two astronauts from each three-man crew landed in the Lunar Lander, while the command-module pilot continued to orbit the Moon until the astronauts joined up again for the return trip to Earth.

The crews used their initiative in choosing the precise landing site and deciding what samples to bring back for analysis. Pete Conrad on *Apollo 12* saw that he was about to land in a crater, took manual control of his landing craft, and put it down safely several feet from the edge. The astronauts who did not land experienced for the first time what it was like to be on the dark side of the Moon, separated from the sight of Earth and temporarily cut off from all contact with Earth. Human emotions were challenged as never before, and they felt a disturbing sense of loss.

Memory: The Diary We All Keep

When circadian rhythms are disturbed, either in space or on Earth (through dodging the pull of gravity by being inactive), we not only experience disturbed sleep and feel depressed, but we also experience confusion and loss of memory. Memory consists of every image and every little bit of information we have accumulated, and can recall, from birth. It shapes our feelings, colors our judgment, influences our choices and decisions, guides our achievements, and comforts us in our old age. Oscar Wilde described it as "the diary that we all carry around with us."

In more modern terms, memory is the "databank" from which we expect to retrieve information at any time. Imagine, then, calling on this databank only to find that "the system is down." Or even worse, that some virus has eaten away half the data. Everyone has had the tantalizing and often embarrassing experience of having a word, or somebody's name, on the tip of their tongue but being unable to recall it.

Memory is what makes us who we are. Not much is left when it is lost. That is why it is so important to do everything in our power to preserve it. Research in this area is moving fast and there are claims of drugs, herbs, and nutrients that help to retard or prevent its loss. But forgetfulness is still a problem that seems to come with advancing years, and as yet there is no single anti-memory loss pill. However, as long as we keep our bodies healthy, there is much we can do to keep our brains active and agile.

How the System Works

The Brain's Reservoir of Untapped Power

It is widely held that most of us use only 10% of our brain, though it is virtually impossible to measure this accurately. What is clear is that we all share more or less the same design of brain circuitry. It is also believed that the brain's ability to respond to new challenges, learn, and store new information confirms that it always seems to have spare capacity, however much it is used.

During the 1960s, I remember reading about a class of mentally-retarded teenagers, considered to have the mental age of five or six-year-olds. They were attending a school in Illinois for handicapped children. An inspired teacher set the challenging tasks and taught them at a level appropriate to their chronological age. When they graduated, they achieved scores within the average of their regular high school contemporaries. The lesson learned is that we never use our brain to its full potential.

Attitudes toward the education of those with mental handicaps have certainly changed in the last forty years, with many students falling into this category going on to university and then leading relatively independent lives. A neighbor of mine in California had four children, the youngest of whom had such a handicap. Katrina attended regular schools, rode her bicycle to high school, and later graduated from community college. The earlier in their lives children who are born with brain damage are surrounded by a stimulating environment, the better their chances are of approaching normality later.

The Remarkable Memory of a London Cabby

As with any other part of the body, if the brain is underused, its cells, the neurons, will not respond as they should when we need them. There is plenty of brain capacity for learning, processing, storing, and retrieving information—if we would only use it. London taxi drivers have long been admired for their remarkable knowledge of the city. Aspiring cabbies have to demonstrate mastery of The Knowledge, as it is called—a mental map of every street, alley, one-way system, shortcut, theater, club, and important building in London. It takes at least a couple of years to learn all this.

MRIs (Magnetic Resonance Imaging) of the brains of such cab drivers at the beginning of their apprenticeship and when they finally qualify for their license show that their corpus callosum, a part of the brain that stores memory, actually grows as a result of the challenge. The development of MRI technology has revolutionized our ability to track changes in size and activity of areas of the brain, and to map the parts that have specific functions, such as learning, balance, co-ordination, and emotion.

It's Never Too Late

Towards the latter part of our lives most of us have to live with the consequences of having "used up" a certain amount of our brain power. But it does not have to be so. The brain can learn at any age, though maybe not as fast as it used to. It is therefore very important to keep it stimulated throughout life, preferably with new experiences. Even if areas are damaged by stroke, injury, drug abuse, or tumor, new connections can form to circumvent and compensate for the damaged parts.

Balance and coordination studies carried out in space amazed us at the plasticity—the ability to grow and change in response to new challenges—of the cerebellum. This is the region at the back of the brain that controls the fine-tuning of movements, enabling different parts of the body to move in a coordinated fashion.

The vestibular system, in the inner ear, which senses direction and acceleration and maintains balance, also proved to be responsive to new challenges. Plasticity has now been shown to occur in all parts of the brain—and perhaps most importantly as we age, the part that deals with memory. The absent-mindedness and forgetfulness that trouble so many of us in advancing years may be the result not of aging but of failing to challenge our brains sufficiently.

The Anatomy of the Brain

The nineteenth century pseudo-science of phrenology held that different regions of the brain were responsible for different character traits in human beings. Its practitioners believed that they could "read the bumps" by feeling a subject's head. They claimed they were able to identify from the shape and size of various areas whether that person had criminal tendencies or was particularly endowed with such qualities as combativeness, caution, idealism, intelligence, altruism, the ability to appreciate music, and so on.

This crude notion has long been exposed as a myth, yet somewhere in the beliefs of the phrenologists there lies a grain of truth. Modern science has established that the brain is organized in such a way that different parts do indeed have specific functions. The marvel is that if one area fails, as can happen due to stroke, its role can be partly taken over by another part of the brain.

All the characteristics we think of as being uniquely developed in humans are centered in the *cerebrum*, or forebrain. This, the largest part of the brain, is made up of two hemispheres, covered by the *cerebral cortex*—about one-quarter inch of deeply grooved, folded, and convoluted "gray matter" formed of neurons, or brain cells. The folding is a way of packing as much surface area as possible into the space available. The greater the surface area, the more room there is for the growth of a network of connections between cells.

Each hemisphere is further divided into four lobes by deep grooves. While the lobes do not appear to be exclusively concerned with specific tasks, there seems to be a fair degree of specialization. Such functions as speech, memory, imagination, intelligence, emotion, and anticipation are primarily the concern of the *frontal lobes.*

Hearing and the sense of smell are located in the *temporal lobes*, those at the sides. The *parietal lobes,* at the top, control touch, while vision is dealt with by the *occipital lobes,* at the rear.

The left hemisphere controls movement on the right side of the body, and vice versa. The right hemisphere seems to be primarily responsible for insight and imagination and for recognizing patterns and shapes, while the left hemisphere specializes in such aspects of mental activity as language, rationality, and number skills.

The two hemispheres do interact, and if some kind of injury causes one to fail in its tasks, the other side can compensate and take over these tasks, provided the damage is not too severe. Between them lies a thick band of nerve fibers called the *corpus callosum*, acting like a bridge that connects the two halves of the brain. Behind and below the cerebrum lies the *cerebellum,* the control center for muscular activity, balance, and co-ordination.

The *hippocampus*, a small seahorse-shaped structure, forms two ridges of tissue within each of the halves of the brain, in the floor of the brain's cavity. Without it, learning and short-term memory are impossible. At the base of the brain, the *hypothalamus* controls the internal activities that keep our bodies running without conscious thought. Among these are the control of body temperature, the release of hormones, the regulation of the digestive system, and the repair of wounds. On either side, the nearby *thalamus* is a kind of junction box that directs information from the senses to the cerebral cortex. These signals are not instantaneous: if you stub your toe, it takes about one-fiftieth of a second for the message, and the flash of pain, to reach the brain.

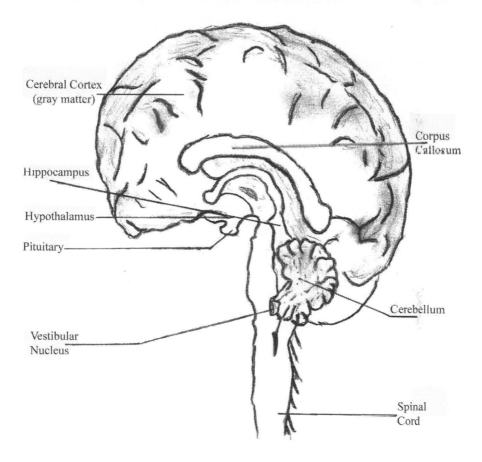

This diagram of the human brain shows the location of key areas in the control of memory, stress, mood, and other functions.

When Brain Cells Die, New Cells Can Be Born

Until very recently, it was believed that once brain cells died, they were never recovered. This has been proven false. Scientist Fred Gage at the Salk Institute for Biological Studies, in La Jolla, California, has convincingly shown in animals as well as in humans that given a stimulating environment, new brain cells develop and that the cells actually *increase* in number. These discoveries change our perspective of what happens to the brain as we age. As with other systems in the body, the loss of brain functions, once thought to be inevitable and irreversible, is now looking both preventable and reversible.

Calling Up Memory…

Scanning by Positron Emission Tomography (a PETSCAN) shows that the prefrontal cortex—the very front part of the cortex—lights up when working memory is recalled.

…and Laying It Down

The process by which permanent memory is laid down depends on the stimulation of neurons and on the strength of the connections between nerve cells. The chemical that transmits signals to them is glutamine, and it can preserve memories for hours or days, but only *short-term memory*. Without the hippocampus, the small seahorse-shaped structure at the base of the brain's cortex, learning, i.e., absorbing new information, is impossible. When first encountered a new item of information may pass back and forth between the hippocampus and the cortex for several weeks before it is finally stored in the cortex.

Permanent storage of information, what we call *long-term memory*, involves the formation of new synapses (links between neurons in the brain) where there is activity, while those neurons that remain unstimulated lose synapses and their nerve endings atrophy.

Research now shows that permanent storage happens during REM (rapid-eye movement) sleep. Disrupting REM sleep also disrupts the formation of long-term memories of events and objects or people. This demonstrates another important connection between a good night's sleep and the ability to remember.

The Three Stages of Memory

As messages flash from the hippocampus to the cortex, memories are laid down in three stages. First comes the *immediate* memory, which can be reinforced if it has any relevance to your life but can be lost in a matter of seconds if your brain decides it is not worth your attention. Then the experience or perception enters your *short-term memory,* from whence it can be recalled several hours later if it is important enough. Finally, given enough reinforcement, it becomes part of your *long-term memory,* which means it can stay with you for the rest of your life. Childhood memories may not be in the forefront of your mind, but they can be triggered by something seemingly trivial—a phrase, a piece of music, or a particular smell. The longest-lasting memories of all are the kinesthetic, or physical motor, memories. Once you have learned to swim, or ride a bike, you will never lose that skill no matter how many years go by without putting it into practice.

The process of laying down memory, then, involves back-and-forth stimulation between the hippocampus and the prefrontal cortex, leading to increased formation of networks between the brain cells.

Education, Education, Education

What this means is that the challenges presented to our memories during life bring about lasting changes in our brains. Studies show that people with better education maintain their memory and other brain functions better when they reach their eighties than their less educated contemporaries. If brain function declines, it usually does so in the eighties.

Scientists believe that people who receive professional training and education are likely to remain more mentally active throughout life. In turn this mental activity results in more dense connections among neurons, and all the brain functions are maintained longer. The researchers who came up with these findings used formal education as their criterion. However, the same principle should apply to self-educated individuals who maintain their curiosity, learn languages and new skills, read, use their brain creatively, and hunger for knowledge. Throughout life, the brain is exposed to all kinds of setbacks, such as injury, drug use, or stroke, which threaten those connections. So the more connections you build and the more learning you do *throughout life*, the less likely you are to suffer crippling losses of memory later.

What Can Go Wrong?

Why Can't I Remember?

There are various degrees of memory loss. If you are in your twenties or thirties, a memory lapse wherein you misplace your keys is not in itself a matter of much concern. As you get older, the other extreme of the memory-loss scale, Alzheimer's disease, becomes a possibility. The forgetfulness that occurs after forty is not Alzheimer's, except in a few cases where it runs in the family. There are some four or five million Americans now suffering from the disease, and estimates of the incidence of Alzheimer's among people over eighty-five range from 25 to 47%. By 2020, the number of Alzheimer sufferers over eighty-five is expected to double as the number of people over eighty-five increases.

About 10% of all Americans over seventy have suffered significant memory loss, but only about half of these cases are due to Alzheimer's. Because women live longer than men, they are more likely to develop the disease. African Americans are also at higher risk, because of their greater propensity to high blood pressure and high cholesterol earlier in life.

Normal forgetfulness affects short-term memory first. It is part of normal aging and can be delayed by keeping the brain stimulated and using gravity in activities that increase brain blood flow.

A rapid change in memory and thinking processes may be a sign of some problem that can be treated, such as thyroid disease, vitamin deficiency, a brain tumor, overuse of medications, chronic infection, stroke, or depression.

Alzheimer's disease is not part of normal aging. It is progressive and at the present irreversible. There is structural destruction of nerve cells in the brain and victims eventually lose awareness of who they are and where they are. This affects the control of what are normally simple body functions, including walking, swallowing, and speaking.

This disease can now be diagnosed accurately enough to distinguish it from normal age-related memory loss. If you seriously think you may be developing Alzheimer's disease, see your doctor. The battery of tests includes scanning procedures, diagnostic tests in blood and spinal fluid, and sensitive neuro-psychological testing.

Alzheimer's: The Risk Factors

Earlier theories about accumulation of aluminum, lead, or mercury in the brain as a cause of Alzheimer's have been disproved. Dennis Selkoe at Harvard Medical School believes the cause is the accumulation of beta-amyloid, a protein that occurs naturally in the body and which forms dense deposits, or plaques, outside and around the neurons in the brain.

Inside the neurons, a mass of twisted strands or tangles is produced. The plaques and the tangles bring the work of the affected neurons to a complete halt. German physician Alois Alzheimer, after whom the disease is named, first discovered and described the tangles of brain tissue in 1907. The hippocampus, which directs memories to the areas where they will be stored, is one of the first parts of the brain to be attacked.

As we age, all of us accumulate beta-amyloid plaque in the brain, much as we accumulate cholesterol in blood vessels, but we do not necessarily get Alzheimer's disease, because the brain, like the rest of the body, has a repair system.

However, age remains the highest risk factor, because repair systems eventually wear out. Other known risk factors for Alzheimer's fall into three categories: genetic predisposition, damage to the brain, and inadequate stimulation of the brain. They include a family history of the disease, mutations of the genes, injuries to the head, inflammation of the brain, estrogen deficiency, stroke, clogged arteries, smoking, alcohol, and lack of education. The disease takes forty to fifty years to develop, because the brain has many different ways of repairing destroyed brain cells.

It's Not So Much Memory Loss as Slower Retrieval

Normal aging memory loss, as distinct from Alzheimer's disease, still allows you to be perfectly functional even beyond your eighties. And it does not happen to everybody. It involves not so much a loss of memory as a slowing down of memory retrieval. Ten years ago, Dennis Selkoe gave this example: "If you're asked a series of rapid-fire questions, you'll have trouble coming up with the answers. But if you're allowed some time, when you're seventy-five, to come up with answers, you may well be able to answer accurately." Nowadays that age may be more like eighty-five. Given more time, you may still get to the right answers. So what's the hurry?

What Causes the Slowdown?

There are many reasons why recall may be slowed down. You may be taking drugs to reduce blood pressure, and some of these may affect memory. Stress and anxiety are other factors that can start a vicious cycle—the more you worry about forgetting something, the more anxious you get, and the worse the forgetfulness becomes. Reduced blood flow to and through the brain can reduce the efficiency of your memory. Brain cells need oxygen, glucose andother nutrients, all of which are delivered by the blood. Good lung function, healthy red blood cells, and brain blood flow are important in providing adequate oxygen.

Anything that interferes with this delivery system will slow down brain processes. Good brain blood flow also takes away the breakdown products and wastes produced by the neurons. This waste material can damage brain cells if it is not removed. Any disease that affects blood vessels, that makes them narrower or stiffer or clogs them up, will reduce the flow of blood through them.

Cerebral vascular disease, the narrowing or blockage of arteries to the brain and within the brain, is more common in men than in women, making men more likely to suffer stroke. Even a minor stroke that is not disabling will result in the death of brain cells. Almost everyone experiences such small strokes at some time in life, some as early as in our twenties and probably more often than we realize. A slight droop on one side of the face or eye area may be a tell-tale sign. Most of the time we are not aware of them and they go undetected. Their long-term effects are so small as to be negligible unless the brain cells that happen to die are in a critical area.

The Shrinking Brain

There is bad news and there is good news about aging and the brain. The bad news is that the brain shrinks as we grow older. There is more fluid in the ventricles, the chambers in the center of the brain, and in the regions at the top of the brain. There is less white matter which contains the masses of dendrites and axons that sprout from neurons and whose job is to carry and receive messages.

This shrinkage was once believed to be the reason brains slow down with age. It was also believed that lost brain cells were never replaced. The good news is that we now know this is not true. Research is showing that, in addition to the build-up of new connections between neurons, new brain cells are generated every day.

Though these new cells would normally die within weeks, stimulating them by learning new tasks may help them to survive. Fred Gage and Carolee Barlow at the Salk Institute for Biological Studies, in La Jolla, California, found that exercising "senior citizen" mice on a running wheel increased the number of brain cells in their hippocampus, the area linked to learning and memory. Gage also showed that new cell growth occurs in human brains as well. The jury is still out on this issue, but the research shows great promise that between generating new cells and learning how to help them survive, the brain can remain agile well into old age.

What Can You Do about It?

In trying to protect the normal brain from aging, promoting brain plasticity—forming new brain cells and connections—is a good place to start.

Increasing Brain Blood Flow

Anything that stimulates brain blood flow is always good for the brain. Blood transports oxygen and glucose to the neurons, the brain's nerve cells. The oxygen is needed to burn the glucose and so provide the energy to make the proteins the brain needs.

Pilots during high-G maneuvers and returning astronauts during reentry into Earth's atmosphere tense their large muscles, such as those in their thighs and lower abdomen. This helps them preserve their brain blood flow and remain conscious when they have to cope with the higher gravity loads that drain blood from their heads. You can get the same muscle-tensing effect by exhaling forcefully. Women who have experienced childbirth using straining maneuvers will know what this means.

There are many ways of sending more blood to the head. One local senior attributes his youthful looks and agile brain to his daily routine of spending fifteen to thirty minutes every day with his head down and his feet up, using gravity to get blood to his head. No, he does not stand on his head in a yoga posture, though that has also been shown to help. Standing behind his armchair, he leans over the back and works his way down till he can rest comfortably with his head and arms hanging over the seat and his legs resting on the back with knees bent. His grandchildren think he is the neatest granddad and join him in his head-down activity.

You can achieve the same effect by lying face down across your bed and easing forward until you are supporting yourself on hands or elbows until your head droops over the side. Or you can lie on a board tilted downwards so that your head is lower than your feet. Large gyroscopes on which people can ride are available at some fun parks and space museums. A twirl on one is a bit like doing cartwheels. It is a lot of fun too. At the Cosmosphere, in Hutchison, Kansas, participants in the Elder Hostel Astronaut Training Program "for the young at heart" say the gyroscope is a most exciting experience and that they feel great afterwards.

Physical Exercise

Inactivity is a sure way to reduce the flow of blood through the brain and slow down its functions. Gravity pulls blood down to the feet, and by exercising—working against gravity—you can pump more blood up to your brain. But physical exercise does more than just increase blood flow. It also increases the number of blood vessels in parts of the cortex.

Kristine Yaffe at the University of California, San Francisco, says that walking vigorously for just ten minutes a day can keep your mind in top shape. She found that women who walked frequently remembered more and were less likely to suffer from mental decline later in life.

Many similar studies in older people exercising regularly on a treadmill at 3 mph for twenty minutes have shown significant improvements in feelings of well-being as well as in learning and memory. In one study, 5,925 women over the age of sixty-five with no mental or physical problems and who walked regularly were monitored for six to eight years. For every mile walked per day, they reduced by up to 13% their risk of lowered mental functioning. Even moderate exercise—eighteen holes of golf once a week, tennis twice a week, walking a mile per day—has been found to provide some benefit.

Electrical Muscle Stimulation (EMS)

The effects of physical exercise on the brain are due not only to increasing the blood flow. Recent research has shown that an electrical stimulus to nerves that supply the leg muscles slows down degeneration of brain cells and increases their plasticity in healthy older people. Even more remarkable is that similar results were achieved in patients with Alzheimer's disease. How this structural improvement translates into improved function is not yet known.

Estrogen and Testosterone

The female hormone, estrogen, maintains synapses (the connections between brain cells) and helps them to grow. It protects neurons and improves brain blood flow in the regions associated with memory. A study sponsored by the National Institutes of Health, in Maryland, due to be completed in 2007, is assessing the effects of estrogen using a variety of tests on 2,900 post-menopausal women who are on Hormone Replacement Therapy. So far, the findings seem to suggest that taking estrogen pills can lead to improvements in verbal memory, reasoning, and attention span. This may be due to the anti-inflammatory and antioxidant benefits of estrogen. But these benefits must be weighed against the increased risk of breast cancer and cardiovascular disease.

Men do not suffer, as women do, from age-related estrogen deficiency, but researchers are now looking into the possibility that the male hormone, testosterone, may offer some similar protection to neurons.

Diet and Drugs

The brain is well protected from physical injury by the skull and by three tough membranes that have shock-absorbing fluid between them. It is also protected from chemical damage caused by substances such as large foreign protein molecules carried in the blood. But these barriers do not protect against oxidation damage to brain cells.

Anything that we can do to keep neurons well nourished and protect them from inflammation or damage by the rogue molecules known as free radicals is well worth the effort. A diet rich in antioxidants (see Chapter 9, "Managing What You Eat") may help to slow down memory loss and the advance of Alzheimer's disease. This is beneficial for older people in general. Anti-inflammatory drugs such as aspirin have also proven to be of some value to those suffering from injury to the brain.

Drugs that lower the level of beta-amyloid, the protein that forms dense deposits, or plaque, around neurons in the brain are now being developed. One day they may be as common as cholesterol-lowering drugs are now. Drugs that produce an increase in the brain transmitter acetyl choline are already on the market. The first of these was Tacrine.

However, the effect of these latter drugs wears off within months. Perhaps the most exciting news of all in this field is that research into a possible vaccine for Alzheimer's disease is underway. Scientists are finding that some anti-inflammatory drugs, such as aspirin and ibuprofen, help by reducing the inflammation believed to trigger this disease, which has long been regarded as incurable. Inflammation in the brain cells produces free radicals that attack the brain, so antioxidants such as vitamin E, estrogen, and diets that avoid excessive quantities of animal fats and sugar but are rich in antioxidants would be similarly protective.

A low-fat diet, exercise, and cholesterol-lowering drugs like the statins (trade names Lipitor, Zoloft) have been found to improve memory retention by reducing damage to the brain's blood vessels and hence the incidence of repeated small strokes. Robert Green at Boston University, in Massachusetts, studying 2,378 patients who were taking statins to lower their cholesterol found that their risk of developing Alzheimer's was reduced by 79%. Brian Austen at St. George's Hospital, in London, England, who showed that the way statins worked was by reducing the production of beta-amyloid, says, "In the general population, people taking statins to reduce their blood cholesterol, for whatever reason, have a 70% reduced rate for developing Alzheimer's Disease." Statins may also help delay the progression of the disease in patients who already have it.

How to Improve Your Memory

Physical exercise is not the only thing that gets results. Any form of exercise for the brain stimulates brain blood flow. Tackling puzzles, learning to recite a poem by heart, learning a new language, or any other mental activity that demands concentration can bring benefits, but something as simple as making the effort to remember somebody's name can increase the blood flow in the hippocampus. And remember: if the brain does not get enough exercise, the connections and synapses, so important to memory, shrivel and atrophy.

Mental exercises can improve memory, especially verbal memory. Many studies have shown that ordinary activities performed with novelty and variety, and engaging as many senses as possible, can prevent natural decline and build up brain cell connections that help keep us mentally sharp. These activities can be everyday happenings such as doing the crossword puzzle, driving to new destinations, eating unusual foods, taking up new sports or hobbies, making new friends, or learning how to play a musical instrument. The goal is to expose oneself to new information and experiences. The stranger and newer these are, the better they stimulate the addition of new networks to process new memories and to retrieve old ones.

A Work-out for the Brain

Larry Katz at Duke University, in North Carolina, put together a set of exercises he calls "neurobics," designed to build up the all-important nerve-brain cell connections. In his book *Keep Your Brain Alive,* he emphasizes he is not talking about curing Alzheimer's but suggesting simple things we can all do to sustain mental agility and head off memory loss. Two I particularly like are "getting dressed with your eyes closed" and "using your non-dominant arm."

You can invent your own. How about lining up some jars containing a selection of herbs and spices and sniffing them with your eyes shut? How many days will it take you to recognize what each one is? The sooner you start, the better. In the process you will enjoy discovering the world around you.

Old neurons are not beyond being stimulated to grow dendrites—nerve sprouts—to compensate for some of those lost with age. Tapes with mental exercises to boost memory and brain agility are now available through the Internet. Thomas Budzynski at the University of Washington, in Seattle, Washington, has produced one of these "Tools for Exploration," which includes simple math exercises.

Though Katz is careful not to make claims that his *neurobics* can help people with Alzheimer's, Robert Friedland and his group at Case Western Reserve University Medical School, in Cleveland, Ohio, are more positive. They surveyed 193 Alzheimer patients and 358 healthy age-matched controls. The subjects were all in their seventies when the study was completed. The results showed that those who had exercised their brains as younger adults by participating in intellectual challenges such as reading, chess, or jigsaw puzzles were 2.5 times less likely to develop Alzheimer's disease. The risk was increased for those who limited their leisure activities to watching TV.

How to Remember Somebody's Name

Some people are not good at remembering names, and this does not get better with age. When you first meet someone whose name you want to remember, try saying it to yourself out loud, for repeating the name will help it to become part of your memory bank. Make a point of being interested in the person and train yourself to connect the name to something you can use to recall it. Perhaps something about the name will help you to create a mental picture. Think of a Mrs. Mason, for instance, with a hammer and chisel in her hand. The more grotesque the mental image, the easier it will be to recall. If you have met a Gabriel Broadbent, for instance, think of him as the archangel Gabriel, complete with wings but exceptionally broad of build and stooping over.

The House of Memories

We all have different tricks we use to jog our memories. The ancient Greeks were so aware of the importance of memory they had a goddess of memory, Mnemosyne. To remember long lists of items, they built up a mental picture of a house with numerous rooms, halls, shelves, and so on, and placed the objects they wanted to remember in that house. All they then had to do when they needed to remember an object on the list was to walk around the house mentally.

We all use the little verbal reminders we now call "mnemonics." They are useful to remember geographic locations, dates, or events or sequences of instructions, as they are sometimes used in the military. A friend uses the word "PAMS" to remind him of the big cities, west to east, in Australia: Perth, Adelaide, Melbourne, Sydney! Mnemonics could be a formula or a rhyme used as a mental trick or an aid in remembering dates. "In fourteen hundred and ninety two, Columbus sailed the ocean blue." Or to remember what happened to the six wives of Henry VIII, you could use: "Divorced, beheaded, died, divorced, beheaded, survived." Many a poor speller has found "I before E, except after C" to be a great boon. You can be creative and come up with your own, or you can look up the many mnemonic web sites for examples.

Skilled memorizers use such mnemonic tricks too. Studying a group of top performers at the World Memory Championships held in London every year, Eleanor Maguire at University College London concluded they were no more intelligent than a control group from similar social backgrounds. However, they were very different in the way they processed what they needed to remember. Whereas both groups used their right brain, the better memorizers also used their hippocampus, which is important for processing the memory of routes and places.

She found that to do this, they used a mnemonic trick, much like the Ancient Greeks, based on placing facts, such as numbers to be remembered, in different locations along a familiar mental route. They then retraced their steps along the route, retrieving the numbers. This technique worked well with numbers but was not as good when it came to shapes or faces. In a way, you do this when you have misplaced your keys and you mentally retrace your steps, checking where you may have left them.

• Setting It All Down

Many of us have said, "I'm having a senior moment" when describing the kind of memory block that can happen as we get older. But let us not forget that there are also improvements in some kinds of memory. Long-term memory remains quite vivid as we age. This is the time to take advantage of this asset and to write down your personal record. Organize those photographs that have never been put into albums and try to say something about each picture. There are many benefits in getting the words and photographic records of your life experiences together—and in writing stories rather than just telling them around the fire-place.

These activities reinforce your faith in your memory. They stimulate your recall circuits in an organized manner and exercise the brain. You will also have a wonderful legacy, a living document for your family and for future gene rations, showing life and customs at a time in history they may not know much about. Try to recall things like what you ate, your favorite song, how much you got paid on your first job, your best dress, your prom, your parents, the naughtiest thing you ever did, and what you did in your spare time without TV and computers. The written document will be physical proof of your life, with its scrapes, flaws, joys, pains, and humor. Every life and every person is different and special. Writing it down helps you remember how special you are.

Writing things down can also improve short-term memory. Here are some other simple ways to improve memory:

Try to prevent the problems that lead to bad memory—poor nutrition, inadequate sleep, anxiety, frustration, and poor brain blood flow from inactivity. Take your time. Plan ahead. Do not rush into things and get yourself into a state. Do not focus on what you are trying to remember. You must have noticed that if you set aside something you are having trouble recalling, it usually pops up in your mind when you least expect it. What is the worst that can happen if you do not remember something? Will you get punished? Will you feel ridiculed? Only if you cannot laugh it off. So don't be afraid of the consequences of forgetting, and don't lose your confidence.

You cannot remember everything, but this is where making lists comes to the rescue. Most people write down things they want to remember. Birthdays, appointments with the doctor or dentist, and the time to pay bills can all be written on a large, easily-visible calendar. Others tie a knot in a handkerchief or wrap string around a finger to remind them of something they need to do that day.

I have always made lists, mostly as a stress-management tool. I have developed a little ritual of looking at my list and my calendar every morning with my coffee, before I start my day. If you are going to make a list, it is important to look at it at least daily. Crossing out things you have accomplished is very satisfying. Looking at calendar and list at the same time provides a cross-check reminder for that day.

I also do something I was unaware of until my husband once brought it up jokingly in conversation. He calls it my "review/preview." He noticed that after lights out, I would go quiet for a few moments, even if he was talking to me. I was not asleep, because I would shortly resume our conversation. On further probing it became evident that I would rapidly review the day's events and just as quickly scan what was on for the next day. Until he raised it, I had no idea I was doing this.

What was particularly amusing was that on mentioning my quirk, my aunt burst out laughing because apparently my uncle did the same. I do not know how many other relatives had this habit. I do know that it is very useful in mentally clearing the decks for the day gone by, and it is an excellent way to ensure a good night's sleep. It serves as a great naturally memory reinforcement. On the other hand, I did not inherit my uncle's remarkable repertoire of jokes. I make a great audience, because I always enjoy a joke as if heard for the first time. Somehow remembering jokes was not a priority for my hippocampus.

Food for Thought

I leave the last word on the brain and aging to Marjory Stoneman Douglas, the *grande dame* of environmentalists, who died in 1998 at the age of 108. In 1987, at age ninety-seven, she said in *Voices of the River*, "There is nothing inherently wrong with a brain in your nineties. If you keep it fed and interested, you'll find it lasts you very well." It is my belief that being active and working against gravity to get the blood up to your head are the two best ways to keep your brain "fed and interested."

Preventing Damage

Before you adopt a healthier lifestyle and begin to harness gravity as your long-term investment in yourself, there are two musts for success. The two chapters in this section discuss these major prerequisites—"Managing Stress" and "Managing What You Eat."

In space, astronauts are exposed to space radiation and to a multitude of unpredictable stresses. All these risks can be life threatening. Living in near-zero gravity further increases the sensitivity of their bodies to damage. Down here on Earth, we face the same hazards, spread out in less acute form over a lifetime.

The rogue molecules known as free radicals build up in the body as the result of exposure to the sun's radiation, poor diet, and unmanaged stress. They attack the walls of cells as well as other cell structures, including their basic genetic material. The damage they cause can lead to a litany of health problems from heart disease to some types of cancer. In addition, poor diet and failure to use gravity properly also cause damage because they send the body's blood sugar levels out of control.

The first step in a successful savings program is to eliminate debt and curb negative habits (compulsive gambling, for example). In the same way, before expecting to enjoy the benefits that flow from using gravity to the fullest here on Earth, it is essential to get rid of any bad health debts. This means protecting the body from damage by sugar and free radicals and dealing with stress by learning to use effective coping skills.

8

Managing Stress

Everybody recognizes stress when they see it, but no one has yet come up with a comprehensive and satisfactory definition of what it is. This could be because it affects different people in so many different ways. A friend passes by in the street without so much as a nod, and to one man this is a trivial event whereas to another it is highly stressful. He broods about the incident day and night, sleeps fretfully, and wakes up with a headache. Stress can cause an entire rogue's gallery of ailments: loss of appetite or compulsive eating, indigestion, diarrhea, constipation, loss of sex drive, difficulty concentrating, increased susceptibility to infection, ulcers, high blood pressure, and the list goes on.

It is my belief that stress is brought on by an event, perceived as a demand, that pushes the body's response beyond its normal comfort limits. *Perceived* is the key word here, for the event itself is less important than the way it is interpreted. *Normal limits* is the range within which various systems in the body fluctuate when we are in good health and in the state of being *well adapted*.

For example, body temperature is considered normal if it fluctuates between 96° F in the morning and 99.9° F in the evening. Outside these limits it can increase or decrease by a couple of degrees before it becomes life threatening. Heat stroke is the result if the body's cooling system breaks down under the stress of very hot summer temperatures. At the other extreme, severe cold can cause death from hypothermia if the body temperature is not speedily brought back within normal limits. The body tries to stay within these limits by shivering when the weather is cold and sweating when it is hot. The normal limits of temperature can also be exceeded in cases of infection. We call this fever.

Our Stone Age ancestors in their caves were no strangers to stress, though their worries must have been somewhat different from the concerns of most people in the modern world. Every day brought a new struggle for survival. They had to find food and shelter, fight off marauding animals, and escape their enemies. Natural disasters could strike without warning—a hurricane, a flood, an earthquake, a forest fire, or a volcano blowing its top.

In today's world we are still engaged in a struggle for survival. Less dramatic for most people, perhaps, but no less real. We all have to provide food, shelter, social status, and a future for our families. Investors need to protect their savings from the vagaries of the stock market, and many employees live in fear of being laid off. People in the *senior* bracket may dread loneliness, burglary, the cost of medical care, loss of independence or their home, and internment in a nursing home until they die. In some countries, people live under the daily threat of a terrorist attack. In others, volcanoes still erupt, and earthquakes can still devastate entire regions.

How we respond to stress depends on us rather than on the event. The key to managing stress is the ability to adapt, to sway with the punches, to be "responsive to change." The first factor to take into account is how seriously you perceive the event as a threat to your physical and emotional well-being. The second is the degree to which you can do something about it. If you do not learn how to manage stress, it can be a killer. And even if it does not kill, it can cause a variety of diseases and bring on signs of aging earlier. All you need do to see its results is to look at photographs of some of the U.S. Presidents of the last fifty years, comparing how they looked before taking office with their appearance after they stepped down.

The Mouse with a Lethal Libido

The tiny male Australian marsupial mouse goes through a two-week frenzy of sexual activity in the spring—a frenzy that ends in death, through stress and exhaustion. He mates with every female marsupial mouse he can find, whether they are receptive or not, dragging them out of their holes if need be, and no sooner finishing with one than moving on to another. During this hormone-driven explosion he has little time to eat, sleep, or even drink. The result is massive physical stress. Odd though it may seem, there may be an evolutionary advantage for the species due to this behavior. With an entire generation of male mice out of the way, the females and their newborn babies will face less competition for food.

How the System Works

How does the brain decide whether something is a stress and whether it is serious enough to warrant a response? Each one of us has a different genetic makeup, has lived through different experiences, and has developed a personal database of memories and attitudes. Faced with a new and possibly threatening experience, we draw on this database. If the demand on our resources is predictable, the brain says, "I am familiar with this. What's more, I am ready for it. There is no need for a stress response." We know that the kids regularly come home from school shortly after school closes at 3 P.M., so their arrival at that time presents no particular challenge. But if the clock ticks around to 4.30 P.M. and they are not home yet, and this has never happened before, an alarm signal rings in the hypothalamus (Greek for lower chamber), a cherry-sized organ that sits strategically in the center of the base of the brain. The hypothalamus sets about mobilizing a stress response.

When Does a Stimulus Become a Stress?

The hypothalamus keeps up a non-stop electro-chemical conversation with the hippocampus, the brain's memory center, which analyzes and evaluates threats, interpreting the information fed into it as either a stimulus or a stress. A stimulus in this sense could be any challenge that activates the entire system sufficiently to keep it primed and maintained within normal limits. Examples are such basic and everyday challenges as getting out of bed, walking, driving, shopping, reading the newspaper, studying, doing a crossword puzzle, or meeting other people. Gravity is such a basic challenge, but increase beyond 1G and it becomes a stress.

Under normal conditions, we are not even aware that such events cause a tiny activation of the stress-response system. But if a routine challenge calls for a response beyond the normal limits, the stimulus may become a stress. For instance, you can sit up or stand many times a day without feeling any different, but if you attempt to stand up suddenly after a day or two in bed with the 'flu, your heart races and you place your body under stress. You will probably feel dizzy and may even faint.

The entire process of evaluating a threat and responding to it happens in a split second. The brain receives information that something has changed in the surrounding world or the brain itself generates a worrying thought. The hypothalamus then scans the database in the hippocampus. How the hypothalamus responds depends on whether the situation was expected and the degree to which the person concerned believes he or she is in control. The process goes along the following lines:

How Severe Will the Stress Be?

Expected Event?	Experienced Before?	How Coped?	Feel Able to Cope?	Stress Response	Feedback to Data Base
Yes	yes	well	yes	0-low	Positive
Yes	yes	well	not now	high	Negative
Yes	no	no data	yes	medium	Positive
Yes	no	no data	no	high	Negative
No	yes	well	yes	0-low	Positive
No	yes	well	not now	high	Negative
No	no	no data	yes	medium	Positive
No	no	no data	no	very high	Negative

Using this chart you can work out, for example, that if you are expecting an event, such as buying a house and moving, this is not your first move, and your previous experience was a good one, you are likely to handle this move effectively. But if this is your first move or you do not feel able to cope, your brain will register it as an unpleasant, stressful experience.

A stress that was previously handled well may become more stressful if conditions have changed—if, for example a person feels incapacitated by age, illness, sleep deprivation, or feelings of helplessness. Every major failure to cope with stress is fed back into the database, and as a result future responses to a stressful event can produce excessive responses within the system—the sign of an inability to cope. The solution is to learn effective coping skills so that successes replace the failures in the data base.

In Space and on Earth—Be Prepared!

Being prepared can go a long way towards preventing anxiety. The extensive training that astronauts go through prepares them to deal with unpredictable malfunctions or emergencies. They learn everything about their spacecraft: how it works, what can go wrong, how to diagnose the fault and how to fix it, and where and when to seek help. They are physically very fit and, to escape a possible fire or a crash at landing, they practice dashing out of their spacecraft wearing their heavy space suits and running away for 100 yards as fast as they possibly can.

Russian cosmonauts go through training that is every bit as thorough, and its value was demonstrated on February 23, 1997, when technical problems beleaguered their Space Station *Mir*. The lithium perchlorate candles that provided life-giving oxygen were running low, and one exploded. A dangerous fire filled the craft for several minutes with choking smoke, but nobody panicked, the fire was put out, and no one was seriously hurt.

On June 25 of that same year, an unmanned 7.5-ton Progress re-supply ship, using a new docking procedure, collided with the *Mir*, damaging its solar panels and depressurizing the science module. The two Russian cosmonauts and British-born U.S. astronaut Michael Foale had the option of returning to Earth in a Soyuz escape ship. However, they sealed off the module and worked valiantly to restore power to the *Mir* by using the power from the Soyuz. There was no loss of life and the *Mir* was saved.

On Earth, the same preparatory rules apply. Fear brought on by unfamiliar sounds during the night or some unknown person knocking at the door brings on a stress response. The feeling can be overcome or reduced if measures are taken to control the situation. Your peace of mind is less likely to be disturbed if you have a good security system, have access to a phone to call for help, and do not open the door to strangers.

By preparing carefully and being well informed, you can take the tension out of many situations. Knowing as much as you can about your subject and about your audience will reduce the stress of public speaking. Finding out about your potential employer before you go for a job interview, anticipating the questions you might be asked, preparing a well-laid-out résumé, and having hand-written material or well-organized visuals for a presentation will boost your confidence and reduce stress. All are essential for success.

"Fight or Flight": How the Brain and Body Respond to Stress

Over millions of years of evolution, human beings have developed what is known as the "fight or flight" response. For our remote ancestors, these were the only options. Coming face to face with a saber-toothed tiger allowed no time for considering long-term strategies. Adrenaline and other fight-or-flight hormones swept through their bodies, and a burst of physical activity was needed, both to deal with the crisis and to clear these hormones from the bloodstream once it was over. We, however, do not always have the opportunity to respond to stress in a physical way. An employee who has just been fired may feel like punching his boss in the nose, but the impulse is usually restrained. In the days when the Japanese were considered the source of all wisdom in business management, some big companies kept life-sized blow-up figures of top management in a basement gym. Overstressed employees could work off their frustrations by punching and kicking the replica of the boss and then report to work calm and composed. The Japanese also have a tradition of being able to verbally unload on their superiors, when drunk together, without repercussions the next day.

Sportsmen and sportswomen, of course, are able to work off an adrenaline surge by running hard, whacking a tennis ball, or doing whatever their sport demands. Without that surge, sometimes referred to as butterflies in the stomach, they would not perform at their best. Actors call the adrenaline surge stage fright. They can be paralyzed by it or use it to improve their performance. Harold Macmillan, Prime Minister of Britain from 1957 to 1963 and a redoubtable debater in the House of Commons, had stage fright so badly that he was often physically sick before making a major speech.

The point about stress is to use it, not be paralyzed by it.

When Stress Hormones Go on the Rampage

The results of the fight-or-flight response are highly visible, but inside the body the process is extremely complex. As soon as the brain identifies a threat as serious, the hypothalamus activates two parallel systems that prepare the body for action: the sympathetic nervous system and a network of hormones, transported in the blood. The sympathetic nervous system sends a stream of electrical and chemical messages to all parts of the body that help prepare the body for action. A power-packed cocktail of hormones—epinephrine (adrenaline) and norepinephrine (noradrenaline) are only two of them   surges through the body.

In a split second, your muscles tense. You feel more alert. Your blood pressure rises. Your heart pounds faster and your blood is enriched with oxygen because you are breathing faster. The pupils of your eyes dilate to take in more light, increasing peripheral vision. Appetite, digestion, and reproduction are inhibited—all of them functions that are not needed for a swift response to stress. Vestiges from our cavemen ancestors are still present in this response. The body hair rises to make us look more threatening. The blood clots more easily to reduce bleeding. And sweating increases, making the body more slippery and tougher to grab.

What happens at the hormonal level to produce this state of hyper-readiness? At the same time as the sympathetic nervous system goes into action, the hypothalamus sends its own hormone, CRH (Corticotrophin Releasing Hormone) to the pituitary, the master gland of the body, to call the hormone network into action. The pituitary hormone ACTH (Adrenocorticotropic Hormone) stimulates the adrenal glands to put out hormones that preserve the body's salt and water, vital to survival. One of these, cortisol, breaks down proteins into amino acids, which are carried in the blood to the liver where they are converted into glucose for energy. Adrenaline steps up your metabolic rate and instructs the liver to break down fats into fatty acids for fuel and to convert starches into glucose for quick energy. Cortisol also diverts glucose fuel to the brain, heart, and muscles by cutting down its availability to other organs. It also constricts blood vessels and controls inflammation at wound sites. Yet another task for cortisol is to ensure that no energy will be wasted, so it suppresses the immune system. Cortisol has been much maligned, called a bad or killer hormone. But it only deserves these negative descriptions when the body puts out excessive amounts, as in cases of unmanaged stress.

The pituitary gland pours out endorphins, the body's own opium-like pain-killers. Endorphins and adrenaline are responsible for the well-known emotional "high" that accompanies excitement. It is because of them that a person injured in a fight, the victim of a car accident, or a soldier wounded in battle may feel no pain when the blow lands, the leg is smashed, or the shrapnel strikes, and only feel the excruciating pain after the stress has subsided. Stress hormones also improve memory, allowing the result of the experience, including a record of how well we coped, to be imprinted in the databanks of the hippocampus.

When the Emergency Is Over

In most cases, the body has its own highly effective way of turning off the stress response tap once the emergency is over. High levels of cortisol and endorphins feed back to the hypothalamus to inhibit further CRH production, bringing the response cycle to a close. This is what engineers call negative feedback. Low levels of cortisol increase CRH production and high levels turn it off.

The Thrill Seekers

It is part of the human makeup to deliberately seek the high that comes when stress hormones race through the body. For a baby, the thrill may come from defying gravity by taking its first steps. As we grow up, it may be getting behind the wheel of our first car, revving up a powerful motor bike, taking a ride on a roller coaster, bungee jumping, sky diving, surfing, skiing, or snow boarding. Why, from a very early age, do we all enjoy being scared by horror movies? This is a way of seeking the high without exposure to real danger. Any physical challenge, from mountain climbing and cave exploring to walking 60 miles to raise money for a charity, brings its own physical and emotional reward. It is by seeking new challenges that we push our limits. My latest adventure was learning how to ride a bicycle at the age of sixty-five!

Some go beyond mere thrills and actually risk their lives. Evel Knievel used his motorcycle to perform incredible stunt jumps. Chuck Yeager broke the sound barrier in an airplane, and Yuri Gagarin was the first human to venture into space. The list of people who have pushed out the barriers is endless. Holger Ursin, at the University of Bergen, in Norway, did a classic study with volunteers recruited to parachute jump out of an airplane. On the first jump, the subjects showed a massive stress response. It diminished with each successive jump. As the sense of accomplishment and control grew, so their fear subsided and their sense of elation increased. Thrill seeking challenges our limits. The physical feat is perceived as a stress, and the body responds to this stress, until the brain learns that the threat is controllable.

One of the greatest thrills of all is to leave the bounds of Mother Earth. Many of us as children gazed at the stars, wondered what lied out there, and dreamed of going to the Moon and beyond. Thousands have applied to train as astronauts or cosmonauts over the last forty years, though very few have been selected. Those who have flown in space are enraptured by their experience. Suddenly liberated from the pull of gravity, they entered a realm of euphoria. They looked down at Earth, admired its beauty, and felt awed by our smallness in the grand scheme of the universe. Those who landed on the Moon had an even more special experience. But those who circled the Moon also felt a sense of loss and depression when they were on its dark side. They could no longer see Earth and felt separated from it. Suddenly, thrill had turned to stress. But why do all astronauts want to keep going back into space? U.S. astronaut John Blaha, who commanded *Columbia* in the STS-58 Spacelab Life Science Mission (SLS-2) that orbited Earth in 1993, called going into space "a buzz." French neurologist Jean-Didier Vincent calls it an "addiction." Are thrill seekers addicts? They may well be. Certainly, the brain networks and chemical transmitters involved in addiction are the same as those involved in the stress response.

What Can Go Wrong?

The brain is bombarded every waking minute with information that demands decisions. What needs doing in the garden? Is that car in front about to turn left, and what do I need to do about it? How am I going to deal with my angry neighbor or my son's disappointment because I did not make his baseball game?

Too many of these demands can become overwhelming, especially if poor health has slowed us down. Too few can lower the overall sensitivity of the response system. If the response to stress is inadequate at one extreme, or excessive and sustained at the other, it can result in a variety of diseases. Which disease one gets depends on such factors as genetic predisposition, diet, and activity levels. If, for instance, there is a history of high blood pressure in your family, a high-salt diet coupled with stress will bring this complaint on sooner, whereas a low-salt diet and an active life may prevent it from ever happening.

The Fear of Losing Control

Research that measured hormone responses in medical students taking exams has shown that every individual has a characteristic stress response, a kind of hormone fingerprint. This profile may indicate that a person is likely to suffer such problems as heart disease, diabetes, or auto-immune disease at a later age—or that he or she is likely to be free of them. Typical behaviors often go with the profile.

Myer Rosenman and Ray Friedman, two San Francisco cardiologists at the Mount Zion Medical Center, classified persons most likely to have a heart attack as Type A after they noticed a lot of wear on chairs in their waiting room not too long after the chairs had been reupholstered. However, the fabric was worn out only at the front edge of the seat, whereas the rest of the seat looked brand new. They concluded that since most of their patients had suffered a heart attack, or were good candidates for one, sitting on the edge of the seat revealed something about their personalities.

Further analysis showed that Type-A patients were always competitive, achievement oriented, and pushed for time. Fear of losing control in their lives was a major threat. Their calmer patients, classified as Type B, did not wear out the fronts of their chairs. They were quite happy not being busy and found that pressure at work was stressful rather than stimulating. Type-A subjects were stressed when they were deprived of work. Type Bs are those with many outside hobbies and interests who are more likely to adapt to retirement and enjoy it, whereas Type As are those most likely to drop dead shortly after receiving their watch.

We hear much about job stress. In the workplace these days, much more is expected from fewer people. Long hours, information overload, less personal interaction, and a stream of e-mail every day—many unnecessary because they come from colleagues down the hall—have become common features of everyday working life. Type As may thrive in this high-pressure environment. Type Bs feel swamped, angry, and frustrated. We recognize Type As as workaholics. Workaholism is a form of addiction.

The Baseline and Daily Rhythms

As with other bodily functions, the hormones that respond to stress fluctuate—rise and fall according to a daily rhythm—within a range of normal limits. The baseline sets the middle of this range. Anything that alters the baseline, alters normal limits or the rhythmicity of these changes, will affect a person's responsiveness to stress. For instance, the stress hormone cortisol peaks before we wake up in the morning. It then decreases throughout the day and remains very low in the evening and into the night unless some stress-provoking event causes a surge in production.

Both the high in the morning and the low in the evening are important for the health of the system. Lower morning levels than the average are often found in inactive individuals, in the elderly, in children living in institutions, and in people with post-traumatic stress disorder, a condition affecting those who have suffered severe emotional trauma from such causes as combat, crime, or natural disaster. Mary Carlson, at Harvard Medical School, studied the children in Romanian orphanages. She found the best performers in motor and mental tests were those with the highest morning cortisol levels, whereas high levels at noon and in the evening were associated with poor mental and motor performance.

Reduced activity in continuous bed-rest is associated with a lower level of cortisol in the blood if the participants see staying in bed as an opportunity for relaxation, and with higher levels if they view it as confinement and helplessness. This is a good example of how the perception of the same condition may or may not result in stress.

In both bed-rest and spaceflight, the adrenal gland gradually becomes less sensitive to ACTH, the pituitary hormone that regulates it. As a result, more ACTH is needed to generate the appropriate response from the adrenal. In bed-rest, this reduced sensitivity takes fourteen to thirty days to develop and it is restored twenty days after subjects get out of bed again. Decreased adrenal responsiveness is common in permanently inactive individuals, including those made inactive by spinal-cord injury. Such reduced sensitivity has long been known to occur as people grow older, but it is most likely the consequence of gradually decreasing activity over a lifetime, rather than of age itself. As with other systems, using gravity to stay active in ways large or small keeps the stress-response system tuned.

Stress in Space

Decreased levels of cortisol would be expected in spaceflight as well, because the gravity stimulus is miniscule. There is no body weight and no sense of acceleration during the flight to stimulate cortisol secretion, as happens on Earth. The *Gemini 7* astronauts, Frank Borman and James Lovell, who in 1965 became the first to fly in space for as long as fourteen days, showed the expected reduced excretion of this adrenal steroid during the flight. Shuttle astronauts had more living space but had to share it with as many as six others, which meant there was very little privacy, causing increased stress and cortisol levels.

The workload on a Shuttle mission is heavy, and the spacecraft noisy. Sleep can be fitful and loved ones are far away. Astronauts endure the helplessness of being controlled from the ground. At times, being in close quarters brings on friction with fellow crewmembers. An unpredictable malfunction, the loss of power, or a crisis such as the fire on *Mir* can be a challenge to the best of them. However exhilarating the view of Earth from space is, the sense of danger is ever present. As the *Challenger* and *Columbia* disasters so tragically demonstrated, exploring the secrets of the universe can be a perilous enterprise. There is no doubt that astronauts with their different personalities view their missions differently. Some may respond excessively to stress in space while others will not. For privacy reasons, data about individuals is not available.

Who's In Charge, You or Your Hormones?

Hormones are blamed for many things: a sudden change of mood or a flare of anger, lack of energy or its opposite, hyperactivity, over-eating or anorexia, depression, lack of interest in sex, a constant, nagging feeling of anxiety. "It's not me, it's my hormones," people will offer as an excuse. But hormones pour into the bloodstream on instructions from the brain, and what the brain has ordered into action, the brain can bring to a halt—or at least slow down.

There is an easily learned technique of willing your heart rate or your blood pressure to come down that is not the restricted province of hermits and holy men on the banks of the Ganges. Herbert Benson, in his book *The Relaxation Technique*, was the first to outline in simple terms the beneficial effects of using mind-over-body techniques to help you relax in order to lower the heart rate or blood pressure.

Deciding that you are in charge of your body is the first step to preventing damage due to stress. Another technique, biofeedback, involves the use of equipment that allows you to see on a screen what is happening to your heart rate or blood pressure. Simply concentrating on the figures and willing them to come down is sufficient to bring them down. Some people can do this in just one lesson. Pat Cowings, at NASA's Ames Research Center, in California, trains astronauts to control space sickness by using biofeedback information. A rising heart rate, increased body temperature, and cold, clammy hands are all warning signs that nausea is on the way.

Before a spaceflight, the astronauts are asked to sit in a chair that produces these symptoms when it is made to spin rapidly. By watching the result on a screen, the astronauts learn to control a function that is not usually consciously controlled. The technique has notched up a number of successes. But Cowings encountered a dilemma with Japanese astronaut Mamoru Mohri, who flew in 1992 on *SL-J*, the Japanese-sponsored Shuttle mission. The Japanese place heavy emphasis on politeness, and from an early age they are brought up to bow and to say *"hai!"* to acknowledge commands. But on the rapidly spinning chair, a nod is practically guaranteed to bring on nausea and vomiting. Cowings explained that during the test she would call out information to him, but on no account was he to nod. But tradition has a powerful hold over the mind. Every time Cowings issued an instruction, Dr. Mohri acknowledged it with a *hai!*, accompanied by a nod!.. becoming nauseous as a result.

Sensitivity to Stress

Probably the most critical factors in determining how an individual will respond to stress are genetic predisposition and early childhood experiences. Seymour Levine's classic experiments at Stanford University, in California, almost fifty years ago emphasized the importance of early experiences. Infant rats that were handled frequently grew up to be more adventurous and inquisitive, whereas their siblings that were not handled kept to the corners of the cage and showed signs of timidity when they became adults. These and later experiments showed that handled animals also have a lower response to a stressful event and lose fewer cells in their hippocampus (the brain's memory center) with age than those deprived of touch when young.

Exposing the mother rat to stress during pregnancy has also been shown to affect the behavior of the offspring. Although such experiments cannot be carried out in a controlled manner in humans, it is not unlikely that stress during pregnancy can have a profound effect on both mother and child. It probably also tips the scale in the direction of post-partum depression, a form of depression that sometimes afflicts mothers after childbirth.

The Need for Recovery Time

Once the stress response has been turned on, it takes time for the body to recover. Allowing adequate time has an important bearing on the way we manage the next stress that comes along. Some everyday stresses can cause greater responses than others and so need more recovery time. It may take only an hour or so to calm down after being agitated because you had too many things to do and were interrupted by irritating telephone calls. But if you have just narrowly avoided an accident while driving, you may be so shaken up that it will take at least a day to recover. The recovery time for somebody who has actually been in an accident, even if they suffered no physical injury, may be as long as a week.

Given a long enough interval between repeated bouts of the same stress, such as riding a bicycle on unfamiliar streets, the response gradually diminishes as we learn or adapt. Given enough time, a human being can adapt to almost anything. However, adapting to one kind of stress does not mean adapting to all stresses. Adapting to the new cycling route does not transfer to other stressful situations, such as starting a new job, and certainly does not help much with your next visit to the dentist.

Bearing this in mind, it is easy to see how a barrage of stresses at frequent intervals can interfere with the ability to adapt, resulting in over-reaction to the next stress. Highly emotional people and others who do not know how to manage their stress tend to overreact. As we get older, we need even more time to recover than we did earlier in life. Managing our time, allowing "free time" between our planned activities for unforeseen events, is the simplest and one of the best stress-management techniques we can use.

We Generate Our Own Stress

So much of the stress we suffer, we generate ourselves. On entering my class of engineering students at Stanford to give a lecture on stress in the late 1970s, I would, as an aside, let a few know about a car in the parking area with two flat tires. Unlikely a story as that seemed, the news spread in a flash and most of the students were on their feet rushing to the door. They were reacting without any further information, assuming they were the victims. I would then ask them to sit down. "One hour will make no difference to the tires." Some students looked resigned, while others twitched restlessly.

Ten minutes into my talk, those who were listening had figured out what my car-tire story was about. The rest were pouring out stress hormones. They were flushed, breathing hard, anxious, and ready to pounce as the clock struck, not able to hear a word of what I was saying—perfect examples of the point I was trying to get across. It did not matter what information I had provided: it was the way it was processed by each individual that determined whether it was stressful or not. How realistically we interpret and evaluate a threat determines how much of a stress response is produced.

The hormone products of the stress response can bring on many mental disorders if they are present in excess or are circulating in the body too long. Cortisol, for instance, amplifies fear-related behavior. Fear is necessary in the initiation of the stress response, but unfortunately the brain can generate fear without a genuine reason, bringing on a stress response that is unnecessary, inappropriate, and counterproductive. People described as "stressed out" are commonly suffering from self-generated stress. They produce high levels of all the stress hormones, leading to anxiety, feelings of guilt, worthlessness, hopelessness, and helplessness.

Depression

Depression is one of the most pernicious and widespread psychological disorders, and it is exacerbated and sometimes brought on by self-generated stress. It can make people sleep too much or not enough, lose or gain weight, accumulate abdominal fat, have problems in their sex lives, and lose interest in life itself. Sometimes it ends in suicide. There are 17 million diagnosed depressed persons in the U.S., and probably many more who are not diagnosed and never receive treatment. The higher levels of stress hormones in depression increase heart rate and blood pressure and may cause blood to thicken, possibly triggering heart attacks. Both coronary artery disease and osteoporosis have been associated with depression. These conditions are not too surprising, since depressives are by the nature of their disease inactive people. Bone loss, heart disease, and depression are especially common in inactive elderly people.

Medical scientists have not yet discovered exactly what happens, but it is established fact that depression can make an existing disease worse. To complete the vicious circle, the disease itself will usually deepen the depression.

Coping with Stress

Stress has come to have negative connotations, but it is absolutely essential for survival. Without it, the body would not be able to maintain homeostasis—the state of chemical equilibrium reached within the body. The body needs small, frequent, manageable stimuli that provoke the stress response in order to keep it in balance. Stress management does not mean abolishing all stress from our lives; it means finding ways to cope with stress levels that would otherwise harm us. When well managed, stress can be beneficial.

Different people use different physical, mental, emotional, or behavioral mechanisms to prevent, turn off, or contain the stress response. But not all ways of coping are of equal value. *Effective coping* means controlling the event and keeping the stress response within manageable limits. Solving a problem, a successful experience at work or resolving a difficult dilemma in a personal relationship are all examples of effective coping.

Believe You Can Do It

Believing you can control a situation is the first step towards actually doing so. This is as true for animals as it is for people. Mice given an electric shock develop ulcers. But if they learn that pushing a lever can terminate the shock, their ulcers go way down. They continue to get fewer ulcers even if the lever is completely disconnected from the shock device and the shocks still come through despite their efforts. The opposite happens, too. Guinea pigs placed in a box in which histamine is sprayed get an asthma attack. They then continue having asthma attacks every time they are in the box, even when no histamine is present.

Stress? What Stress?

In my early days with NASA in the 1960s, I met the airplane test pilots at Dryden Research Center, in Southern California. They were about to start testing concepts of a remotely-piloted vehicle (RPV) flown by a pilot on the ground. However, they did not want to crash this one-of-a-kind item of expensive experimental technology, so there was still a pilot in the vehicle who would take over only in an absolute emergency. I thought this was a great chance to measure stress levels. After explaining that I needed a donation of urine from them, in order to measure stress hormones, they stood up and thanked me, and one of them, Bill Dana, asked, "Little lady, why would I want to know if I was stressed?"

As I headed back home empty handed, I realized I had just received my first lesson on how these extraordinary men face death in their jobs. To be successful at what they do, they must believe they are in control.

Worrying whether they were stressed would interfere with their performance.

Several years later I had the opportunity to measure cortisol in a group of men doing what anyone would think is an extremely stressful job. Three pilots flew U-2 planes three times a week at NASA's Ames Research Center, in California, for an ecological survey program. Fifteen years earlier they had been flying spy missions, as Gary Powers had. Each flight now lasted about 2 hr 45 min. At altitudes beyond 60,000 feet, they wore pressure suits and breathed 100% oxygen. Their feet were cold and their heads got hot as they got closer to the sun. They had to recalculate and re-adjust fuel distribution in the plane to avoid stalling and were pleased if they stalled only about eight times per flight. To top it all off, they had to photograph the terrain using a camera attached to a periscope device through a hole in the bottom of the plane. That was the primary reason for their being up there.

A highly stressful experience, one would have thought. But not only was their cortisol not increased, it was even lower than when they were on the ground. The only time one of them showed a stress response was on a day when there were strong crosswinds and a downdraft on landing. This reinforced the evidence that learning to believe they were in control meant they were not simply reacting to stress but actively suppressing the stress response.

It's Good to Talk

The power of the psychological element is frequently ignored in clinical studies. For more than twenty years it had been generally agreed that bed rest causes stress, since more of the stress hormone, cortisol, was measured in the urine. But our research provided new clues into ways of reducing stress—and a fascinating slant on the differences between the sexes. In 1982, we did our first head-down bed-rest study using women volunteers. To my surprise, I found that after a rise on the first day, due to being in a new and unusual environment, their cortisol levels showed no further increase, and even went into a slight decline. With men it stayed high.

When we selected volunteers to take part in our studies, we always gave them a detailed briefing about exactly what would happen. This was taped, and we did not deviate in practice from what we told them. On the morning we briefed our first women volunteers, I distinctly remember the hubbub of voices in the conference room. Sixty women, from all walks of life and who had never set eyes on one another before, were socializing and chatting up a storm. With men, we had invariably met a quiet and muted audience.

The eight women finally selected were mostly professionals—an attorney, a nurse, a radiation technician, and a travel agent among them. They came in with definite plans about how they would spend their time and what goals they expected to accomplish. They also talked a lot about various aspects of the study. This was distinctly different from the behavior of our male volunteers, who did not talk about their feelings unless asked to, and even then very reluctantly. Mostly, men tended to talk about sports and money.

With the next study with men, I tried a little psychological experiment. I quietly asked the few men who had taken part in previous studies to act as unofficial mentors to first-timers. Then I paired them up in rooms with the rookies we had selected. No increase in cortisol excretion was seen in any men this time—nor at any later time. The indications were that they had reduced their stress levels simply by venting their concerns—just as the women had done.

Facing Up to the Challenge of Age

The challenges that face us typically change with age. The ability to keep some sense of personal control is eroded by other peoples' attitudes, as well as by physical slowing down. Something as minor as the need for reading glasses can be a major blow to one's independence. It can affect the ability to drive, for one thing. Even more serious are the three most likely events that come with getting older—retirement, loss of a significant other, and relocation.

Relocation, to a nursing home in particular, is with few exceptions a one-way street. Judy Rodin, now president of the University of Pennsylvania, did some very important research when teaching coping skills to the residents of a nursing home. She worked with them and the staff to reduce the tendency of elderly people to attribute their shortcomings to their physical state. For example, they were told that the floors of the nursing home were very slippery because they were tiled to keep them clean. Even young people could slip on them. In this way, the residents would refocus their own thinking and stop blaming weak knees or poor coordination, passing the blame instead to an environmental factor. Residents in nursing homes often have very high cortisol levels, similar to those found in patients suffering from depression. In this case, acquiring coping skills and learning how to perceive that they had greater control of their lives reduced their cortisol levels to normal and improved their general well-being.

Another successful approach to developing coping skills that you can try yourself was developed by Florence Clark at the University of Southern California.

Although she calls it "occupational therapy for independent older adults," it is essentially comprised of coping skills that are tailored to the individual. She studied 361 subjects over the age of sixty for several months. One example was "an eighty-year-old woman who was depressed, spent most of her days in bed or watching television. She rarely ventured out of her building because she was unfamiliar with public transportation and was afraid of falling when taking that first 'big step' to climb aboard a bus."

The therapist identified the problem as the size of the step. She provided a step to practice on that was of similar height to that from the street onto the bus. She also helped the subject with her first trips out on the bus and then directed her to try it on her own. The woman reported later that she felt healthier and regained some sense of independence. Other persons of the same age in the study who were given equal time and attention for social activities, such as games, movies, or craft projects, showed no improvement.

Fake Solutions

Ineffectual coping, however, is by far the most common way the majority of us appear to handle life's stresses. We each develop favorite ineffectual coping behaviors that do not work properly because they are not aimed at the cause of the stress itself. In the late 1960s, I was studying how the brain and the pituitary-adrenal system respond to various types of chronic and acute stress. At the same time, my colleagues at Stanford University, in California, Bob Conner and Seymour Levine, were doing research into aggressive behavior.

In their research, a rat receiving a mild electric shock to its feet would jump and lick its paws. A pair of rats receiving the same shock resorted to attacking each other, presumably thinking the other guy did it! The number of attacks was used to measure aggressiveness. I asked if I could measure the stress responses in these animals, fully expecting that fighting would add further stress to the stress of the electric shock. But when the animals had another rat to fight, they showed much lower stress hormone responses than when they only got a shock. After doing everything we could to exclude other interpretations, we concluded that the fighting behavior represented a way of coping. It was ineffectual, since fighting did nothing to change the duration of the shock or relieve its intensity.

We humans indulge in many inappropriate coping behaviors to make ourselves "feel better": bursting out in anger, smashing dishes, physically or verbally abusing a spouse, fighting people who have annoyed us, daubing a wall with graffiti, damaging public property. However, any benefit from these behaviors is slight, while the harm to ourselves and those around us can be huge. Such behavior can place an intolerable strain on family relationships and put at risk one's job and financial independence.

It can also be damaging to health. Anger and hostility are documented killers, increasing the risk of heart disease. Research has shown that angry people have an increased output of stress hormones, causing higher blood pressure and a speeding up of the heart rate. A study of young doctors and lawyers carried out in the late fifties, and followed up twenty-five years later, found that those who had high hostility were four to five times more likely to develop coronary heart disease later in life. What was even more dramatic was that of those who at the age of twenty-four had been assessed as being angry, 14% of the doctors and 20% of the lawyers had died by the age of fifty as compared to 3% of the doctors and 5% of the lawyers in the other group.

Ineffectual coping methods include excessive eating or dieting, smoking, drinking, obsessive exercising, excessive use of health-food medicines and over-the-counter drugs, use of sleeping pills, and use of recreational drugs such as cocaine and a variety of narcotics and/or stimulants. Such "solutions" to the problem of stress can harm both the individual and other people. Any activity that is done obsessively—gambling, playing the stock market, shopping for things we do not want or need, spending hours at a time watching videos or web surfing—falls into the category of false solutions.

Dodging the Issue

Avoiding a problem rather than addressing it—otherwise known as procrastination—is a common example of a *non-coping* behavior. If you put off going to the ophthalmologist or the dentist because you are worried about what the visit may reveal, all you are doing is adding to your stress by conjuring up problems that may be far worse than the facts warrant. During the 2000 Census, many seniors put off filling out their forms, worrying that the information might be misused. An annual avoidance ritual has grown up around the requirement to file income-tax returns—as evidenced by the rush to the post office at the last possible moment.

In its most serious forms, avoidance can result in "freezing," the loss of the ability either to fight or to fly. Sufferers from this extreme form of procrastination will stay in bed or sleep all day, escaping to a fantasy-land staring at the TV or a computer for hours without really watching. An example of non-coping seen frequently these days is "caregivers stress," which especially afflicts the daughters of elderly parents who have Alzheimer's disease or have suffered a debilitating stroke. Because the image the caregivers carry in their heads from childhood is one of their parents taking care of them, they do not cope very well with the role reversal. Some do not cope at all. They do not dare to leave their parents alone and are not willing to hand them over to other caregivers, so they go through social withdrawal, hardly ever seeing anybody outside the immediate family. Stress may also develop because of a neurotic need for control. Caregivers become anxious, depressed, exhausted, and irritable and end up compromising their own health. They need to learn coping skills, to relax and allow others to help and give them time off to recover.

Life Events That Cause Stress

In 1967, T. H. Holmes and R. H. Rahe at the University of Washington, in St. Louis, published a scale of social life events rated by how stressful they were. Their data was extracted from case histories of patients hospitalized for treatment of medical problems—the more severe the medical problem, the higher the score given for the life events the patient experienced during the previous two years. Note that events represent a *change* of some kind. Not all would be necessarily viewed as bad.

If You Want to Lighten the Burden, Share It

Your appraisal of a situation may bring on an emotional response ranging from excitement and happiness to fear, guilt, or anxiety. This in turn influences the choice and the effectiveness of the coping strategy you adopt. Moving house may raise physical concerns of packing, financial worries, and the emotional turmoil of going through and disposing of mementos. All told, the task is daunting and stressful. Do not expect to do it all at the same time and by yourself. Separate each aspect of the move. Organize what needs to be done before you even start and allow plenty of time to accomplish each task. Seek help or advice even if you do not follow it. Others may have creative ideas. Throw a pot-luck party where friends come to do specific tasks around the house. Allow yourself a break to relax or take a walk.

There are stressful life events that are almost beyond management. Jorn Olsen and his team at the University of Aarhus, Denmark, analyzed the records of 21,062 parents who had lost a child. Not surprisingly, they found that the death of a child was even more stressful than that of a spouse. There was a far greater mortality rate among mothers and fathers in the first three years after such a loss. Single mothers were most vulnerable, and fathers who got cancer had a worse survival rate than was average in Denmark. Mothers who lost a child from unnatural or unexpected causes had the highest mortality rate of all.

The Holmes-Rahe Scale

Life Event	Stress Rating
Death of spouse	100
Divorce	73
Marital separation	65
Jail term	63
Death of close family member	63
Personal injury or illness	53
Marriage	50
Fired at work	47
Marital reconciliation	45
Retirement	45
Change in health of a family member	44
Pregnancy	40
Sex difficulties	39
Gain of new family member	39
Business readjustment	39
Change in financial state	38
Death of a close friend	37
Change to different line of work	36
Change in number of arguments with spouse	35
Mortgage over $100,000	31
Foreclosure of mortgage or loan	30
Change in responsibilities at work	29
Son or daughter leaving home	29
Trouble with in-laws	29
Outstanding personal achievement	28
Wife begins or stops work	26
Begin or end school	26
Change in living conditions	25
Revision in personal habits	24
Trouble with boss	23
Change in work hours or conditions	20
Change in residence	20
Change in schools	20
Change in recreation	19
Change in church activities	19
Change in social activities	18
Mortgage or loan less than $30,000	17
Change in sleeping habits	16
Change in number of family get-togethers	15
Change in eating habits	15
Vacation	13
Christmas alone	12
Minor violations of the law	11

Source: Holmes-Rahe, "Holmes-Rahe life-changes scale," *Journal of Psychosomatic Research* 2 (1967), 213–218.

Dealing with Addiction

Research into the relationship between drug addiction and the stress response is opening up huge possibilities for understanding both processes and finding new ways of treating them. Underlying both is the basic need to "numb the pain" on the way to "feeling good."

An important issue in drug dependency is craving—an intense desire to re-experience the effects of the drug. People who have stopped taking drugs or smoking always find that the craving continues long after the habit is discontinued. Research shows that the craving is closely related to the release of the body's own opiates, or painkillers. The drug Naltrexone, which counteracts the effects of opiates such as morphine or heroin, was surprisingly found to decrease the craving for cocaine and alcohol. Exactly how this works is not yet clear, but this treatment provides a new way to help prevent "cured" addicts from relapsing. On the other hand, stress or the release of the hormone CRH, which initiates the stress response, can restore craving. CRH, which also raises anxiety, is increased in the brain of addicts who are attempting to break free from their habit.

Addiction has many forms. It can involve drugs, nicotine, alcohol, overeating, anorexia, bulimia (overeating followed by vomiting) and even compulsive behaviors such as nail-biting, incessant hand-washing, compulsive neatness, or excessive exercising. As with other addictions, these behaviors produce physical withdrawal symptoms when stopped, and often the stoppage is soon followed by a relapse. For example, excessive eaters who go on diets feel deprived, and just like drug addicts they know how easy it is to relapse.

Equally, although exercise is good for you and is needed at all ages, obsessive exercising is an addiction and can be damaging. It is a case of excessive stress. It is not unlike overusing gravity such as the hypergravity that would be experienced by spinning very rapidly on a centrifuge or pulling high G on an aircraft. Male rats living at 2 G have smaller testes and lower levels of the sex hormone testosterone.

Male marathon runners show a reduced production of testosterone and women marathoners often stop menstruating. If they discontinue exercising for any reason, they go through withdrawal symptoms, feeling sluggish, unwell, and depressed. It has been suggested that this may be due to the craving for the pleasurable high from the stress hormones and opioids released by daily exercise. Risk taking and thrill seeking taken to excess may become obsessive or addictive.

The Consequences of Unmanaged Stress

Chronic stress, the cumulative effect of repeated stress bombarding us relentlessly, can take a heavy toll. The stress-response system may no longer be able to shut itself off. Damage is caused by the very hormones and processes that are intended to protect us from danger in the first place. Overreacting to stress makes us more susceptible to various diseases that shorten life. High blood pressure becomes chronic, and blood clots form more readily, increasing the likelihood of a stroke. Increased blood sugar can lead to diabetes. There is an increased likelihood of ulcers and irritable bowel syndrome. The bones lose calcium and become fragile. Joints and skin lose their collagen, so the joints become arthritic and painful and the skin wrinkled. Muscles waste—a symptom that is fairly common in people with chronic stress, and is often seen in the elderly.

Too much of the hormone cortisol can damage neurons, or brain cells, especially in the area of the hippocampus, the structure vital to learning and memory. At first, the effect is reversible as new neurons fill the gaps, but after several months of high cortisol levels, neurons that die are lost permanently. Situations that lead to persistent high cortisol secretion, such as months of depression or exposure to combat, can cause the atrophy of as much as 10–25% of neurons in this area. To put it brutally, too much uncontrolled stress can cause permanent brain damage.

Stress and cortisol suppress the immune system and its ability to defend the body. The body's first defense against injury or infection is inflammation. That is why the first response to a cold may be a red and raw sore throat, and it is why redness and tenderness build up around an infected injury. Immune cells rush to the site of infection to fight off bacteria and viruses to promote healing. Nearly all of us come into contact with some form of infection every day, but because we have a healthy immune response, we rarely contract an illness. Some viruses, however, like herpes, the bringer of cold sores, remain present in our bodies in an inactive state, and at times of stress they can flare up. This has been shown to happen in spaceflight as far back as the Apollo days in the 1960s.

A similar falling off in the immune response has been found in other confined environments, such as polar stations, submarines, hospitals, and nursing homes. With increasing age, the ability of most humans to organize an effective immune response decreases. Elderly people who have to be taken into hospital are much more likely to get pneumonia than younger people, and often with fatal consequences. Harnessing gravity by making a deliberate effort to remain active can keep the immune system vibrant.

Cancer and infectious diseases occur much more frequently in those whose immune systems are run down, and for a cancer patient, handling the stress of the disease is one of the keys to survival. A group of patients with skin cancer who took part in a six-week program where they learned stress management and coping skills and received psychological support increased their chances of survival and showed no recurrence of the disease five or six years later. The support of loved ones, friends, and relations is one of the most effective coping interventions.

A disturbed stress response and excessive inflammation have been implicated in auto-immune diseases such as rheumatoid arthritis, Crohn's disease, and lupus. Auto-immune disease describes the condition in which antibodies manufactured by the immune system turn against our own bodies as if they were attacking a foreign invader. In the case of arthritis, it is joints that are the target. In Crohn's disease, it is the lower intestine, and in lupus, it is mainly the skin and other connective tissue.

What Can You Do about It?

Flying in space is a dangerous occupation. Astronauts go through intensive training to prepare them for the numerous stressful circumstances they are likely to encounter. The basic principles and techniques they learn are incorporated into this section.

• Be Prepared

The astronauts always are. If you are ready to deal with a stressful situation, you are halfway to beating it.

• Learn Coping Skills

The more often you cope well with difficult situations, the more your coping skills increase. Astronauts analyze the coping techniques they have been using and, if necessary, learn how to modify them to cope more effectively with stress. They go through types of wilderness training to learn creative ways of coping in difficult situations. As part of the collaboration with the Russians, one of these involves being parachuted into the Siberian wild in the middle of winter and having to fend for themselves for several days. They need all their creativity to survive and find their way to shelter. This reinforces their self-confidence in their ability to cope.

• Learn to Relax

The support system developed by team building is a major part of astronaut training. On the last journey of *Columbia*, in January 2003, Commander Rick Husband surprised onlookers by praying with the other six astronauts as they embraced before entering the spacecraft to launch. The crew represented different countries and faiths. This was his way of giving them comfort and helping them to relax.

Stretching is a very important component of relaxing, especially as we age and tend to become stiffer. Try to do some gentle stretching every day. Swimming, too, is a great way to relax joints and wash away muscle tension. So is taking a warm bath. Make a ritual of it, using sweet-smelling bath salts if you desire.

The Case of the Stressed-out Astronaut

I remember driving through the gates of NASA's Ames Research Center, in California, early one morning behind a car whose driver seemed to have no neck! "My goodness," I thought, "here is a very stressed man." His shoulders were tensed up right up to his ears, and the back of his neck was very red. As I passed him I discovered, much to my surprise, that it was Al Worden, an Apollo astronaut who had circled the Moon. On reaching my office, I called to find out what was wrong.

"Terrible day, terrible day" he mumbled, "but how did you know?" After I described what I had seen, I suggested he go to the window, take a few deep breaths, and push his shoulders down away from his neck. If he had trouble doing that, I told him to rotate them backwards until he had a neck again. Then drop his jaw open!

It may look foolish, but there is no way you can not be relaxed with your jaw open. You cannot even frown with your jaw open. Try it! Then ask yourself, "Could things be worse?" They always can.

Worden thanked me later. I taught the jaw trick to my NASA colleague Bob Rhome. Sitting across the table at directors' meetings, I would "watch" his blood pressure rise. After catching his eye, I would drop my jaw as daintily as I could. He would promptly reciprocate, trying to hold back a smile. The stress was defused.

The basic relaxation technique is to set aside a few minutes of quiet time. Sit down without slouching, but in a comfortable, relaxed position, hands resting on your thighs. Breathe in deeply through your nose to the count of four, and then exhale slowly through your mouth. Repeat this three to four times. Close your eyes, let your muscles go limp (as well as your jaw), and relax your whole body. Visualize yourself resting in a calm, favorite place. Allow yourself to fully experience all sights and sounds of that calm, beautiful place for a few minutes. When you are ready, take a deep breath, open your eyes, and think of yourself as refreshed and energized. Stretch gently.

• Believe You Can Make a Difference

The brain can perceive the same situation as a threat, a commonplace event, or a thrill, and perception makes all the difference to how the body responds. For instance, pain, which is considered by anyone as a stress, can be relieved either by medication or by a placebo, a substance that contains no active drugs. But for the placebo to work, the brain has to believe in its power. A recent study on the value of arthroscopic knee surgery (the use of an endoscope to inspect the inside of a joint) showed that pain was relieved just as effectively for patients who only underwent placebo procedures as for those who received the full surgery.

• Stop Worrying

You can avoid stressful situations up to a certain point. To prevent sunburn, you stay out of the sun. If you find driving stressful, don't drive at night or during rush hour or on icy roads. Worrying about some impending disaster over which you have no control causes unnecessary stress and anxiety.

When I was living in California, I had to straighten the pictures on my office walls every morning, because small tremors happened all the time. I soon accepted this as a simple fact of life, but some of my neighbors moved away. They were paralyzed with worry about when the next big earthquake might hit. Another classic example of self-generated stress comes from believing rumors and worrying about things that may never happen. During the thirty-two years I worked at NASA, my department was reorganized more than fourteen times. Rumors of pending reorganizations were therefore constantly circulating. Paying attention to them could freeze one's ability to function—as indeed happened to some. Their work and health suffered, and all they could do was to discuss the rumors all day.

• Do Something about It

Most importantly, you should take action. The best action is to remove the cause of the stress, but even a diversion, such as taking exercise, can be effective. Most of the stress we suffer is psychological and therefore manageable. The brain, which initiates the stress response in the first place, should theoretically be equally capable of managing the stress as well.

• Think Before You Act

To make progress in managing stress, you should first pause, count to ten, take a few deep breaths, push your shoulders down, relax your jaw, and analyze what it is that is worrying you. Is there something you can do about it? If not, worrying about it is only a waste of energy.

• Make lists—and Accentuate the Positive

Identifying the real source of a problem and then realistically sizing it up goes a long way towards resolving it. Write down every possible thing that is bothering you. Look at the list, item by item. You will find that you can dismiss some worries as unfounded. Are you worrying about something that may not happen? No amount of worrying is going to change the outcome. Cross it off. Some world event or tragedy you heard about on the news has you worried? Perhaps there is a small way you can help, by sending off a letter or a donation. If you can, do so, and you will feel better. Otherwise, cross it off.

Older people tend to see themselves in a negative light, based on feelings and behaviors they attribute to aging. If they drop something, they are quick to say, "How stupid of me" or "I can't do anything right." Make a list of your positive and negative thoughts or statements—especially the positive ones. "I cannot do anything right" should be challenged by several positive statements of things you always do right. This holds true at any age. Seeing the glass as half full rather than half empty makes for a healthier, happier life.

• Do Something You Can Control

Diverting attention to something you can control is another way of keeping calm. Stewing over how much you lost in the stock market dive of recent years is a waste of energy and can make you feel low. But how much did you really lose when you compare the current value of the stock not with its peak price but with what you paid for it in the first place? And have you the things that really matter—your health, your family, your job, the roof over your head?

• Make Your Goals Attainable

If you have a long-term goal, you are more likely to reach it by taking small, controllable steps. Make sure every day includes one or two things, however trivial, that you are sure you can accomplish. Write a letter, call a friend, or read ten pages of a book. At the end of the day you can look back and say, "I did x and y..." rather than be overpowered by statements like "I have so much to do."

• Reward Yourself

Are you still worried about something and cannot get it off your mind? Reward yourself. Have your hair done. Get a massage. Buy a new necktie or something pretty. Have a glass of red wine (only one!). Surround yourself with pleasant ways of stimulating your senses. Buy some flowers or work in the garden. Sniff some herbs or fresh roasted coffee or even freshly baked bread. An aunt once advised me the way to keep my husband happy was to fry onions or bake cookies at about the time I expected him home. It mattered little if they were not meant to be eaten; the aroma that greeted him evoked a warm welcome.

• Laughter, the Great Healer

Do not forget to laugh. Lee Berk at Loma Linda University, in California, showed that "happy, silly" laughter, in contrast to pretend laughter, reduces stress-hormone levels and boosts the immune system. Best-selling author Norman Cousins brought attention to the health benefits of laughter in his book *The Anatomy of an Illness*, published in 1991. Bedridden and weak, suffering with ankylosing spondylitis, a degenerative connective-tissue disease, he discovered he could only sleep after watching *Candid Camera* and Marx Brothers films. He also noticed he was in less pain. He had been given a one-in-five-hundred chance of recovery, but somehow he eventually did recover, and he attributes it to the healing effects of laughter.

The idea is being explored in a five-year study at UCLA, under the title "Rx Laughter," in which researchers are evaluating the impact of laughter in both healthy and very sick children. Much like Cousins, they are using vintage comedy of Chaplin, Abbott and Costello, W. C. Fields, Buster Keaton, and the Marx Brothers, which is completely fresh to these kids.

Bill Marx, son of Harpo Marx, says of the project, "When you have a sense of humor, you automatically have an option on your view of life." Ronald J. Fields, grandson of W. C. Fields, comments, "Humor is nothing but extreme positive thinking." Psychologist Margery Silver, who collaborated with Tom Perls on *The New England Centenarian* study, observed that centenarians often have a great sense of humor, finding it in ordinary things. She says they found that "laughter is like internal jogging."

• Meditation, Biofeedback, and Yoga

Meditation involves sitting relaxed, breathing gently, and calming the mind by emptying it of thought, concentrating on or contemplating just one thing.

Self-hypnosis uses mental imaging. Try to see yourself in your mind's eye relaxing, sinking into the floor, or wading into warm, soothing water. With this comes mental relaxation.

Biofeedback is a relaxation technique that enables you to lower your blood pressure or heart rate by observing them on a display screen.

Yoga is a helpful relaxation technique that includes breathing and stretching exercises.

Information about these techniques can be found on web sites, your local fitness facility or YMCA, and your local newspaper.

• Have a Massage

Massage, adjusted for age and condition, is being increasingly recognized for its relaxing benefits to the mind and body. Try it with aromatic oils—chamomile or lavender are best—to a background of gentle soothing music. A study in ten healthy adults aged sixty-three to eighty-four published in 1998 in the *Journal of Gerontology* found it brought about an improved immune function, better sleeping and eating patterns, and reduced anxiety and stress hormones. Many nursing facilities now include shoulder, hand, and foot massage once a week. For those who can afford it, whole body massage is very beneficial. It improves circulation to the muscles and reduces muscle cramps and swelling around joints. However, make sure you talk to your doctor first if you have osteoporosis, blood clots, diabetes, cancer, or other conditions the massage therapist needs to know about.

• Don't Forget Prayer

We all pray at one time or another, whether we acknowledge it or not. When we say, "I wish the sun would come out" or "I wish the pain would go away," that is a form of prayer, because it is addressing a greater power in whose goodness and omnipotence we believe. Prayer can be regarded as another form of meditation that can calm, relax, and relieve anxiety. Many people have found comfort in prayer when facing distress, danger, or death.

Scientific research into the links between religious belief, health, and longevity has, however, been controversial. Individuals may draw strength, comfort, and a sense of security from faith in a greater power without being regular churchgoers.

However, congregations of all faiths are an invaluable source of support, especially to those who live alone.

• Manage Your Time

Perhaps the most effective means of reducing anxiety is to manage time effectively. Things we "should do" seem to creep up on us, until they become overwhelming. I have found that my favorite practice of list making comes to the rescue. Writing down what "I should do" is not only a memory jog. When the job has been carried out, I have the satisfaction of crossing it off the list.

At the start of each day, make a mental note of what you would like to accomplish—make telephone calls, exercise, go to the cleaners, pick up groceries, visit a sick friend or an exhibit. Whatever the task is on the list, allow at least fifteen minutes more than you expect it to take. Then you will not become frantic if you start to fall behind. Any time you try telephoning a public company these days, you have to talk to a machine, and you will almost inevitably find that it takes longer than you expected to get through to the person you want.

• Exercise—at Your Own Level

For those able to exercise, the most obvious benefit is the relief of anxiety. People who exercise regularly are calmer, less angry or tense, happier, and better sleepers. Exercise can improve immune function, too. It is particularly effective for people who suffer from low-level anxiety. And it's a lot cheaper than anti-anxiety drugs. However, if you are taking pills, do not give them up without first checking with your doctor.

If you do not already exercise, start slowly. Set a pace that is beyond a shuffle and enough to raise a sweat. Do your exercises standing up rather than sitting down. If all you can do at first is stand up several times, it is a great beginning. The more days a week the better, but start with three times a week, allowing time to recover. Do not expect immediate changes in your anxiety symptoms. You do not get rapid results with drugs either. Do not start out by setting yourself unreasonable goals: that will only increase your anxiety. Wear comfortable shoes and loose clothes, and equip yourself with your favorite music or radio program. As with other stimuli, you are more likely to stick with exercise, and it will be more beneficial, if you vary it. Although most experts agree that aerobic exercise, such as walking, running, or bicycling, is more effective in reducing stress than weight training, opinions now seem to suggest that all forms are beneficial. A University of Manitoba research study found that aerobic or anaerobic exercise of low to moderate intensity lasting twenty to sixty minutes three times a week produced improvements in mood within five weeks.

• Develop a Circle of Support

Surrounding ourselves with other people can also provide protection from the harmful effects of stress. The emphasis here is on support, not just social activities. People who are involved in warm, loving relationships are likely to live longer, healthier lives. Research has even shown that sociable people are the least likely to catch a cold. In contrast to general assumptions, the *New England Centenarian Study* found that instead of being abandoned and alone, centenarians had strong family ties and many close friends. Madame Marie Simrova of Calgary, 103, says she has a strong circle of younger friends "mostly because my contemporaries have died." It gave her the incentive to dress up and look as elegant as she always did. A circle of close friends does not just happen. She worked at developing and keeping these younger friends, and they enjoyed learning from her.

In contrast, social isolation, the stress of being alone without close friends or family, increases anxiety and seems to trigger signals in the body that suppress the immune system, increasing the risk of sickness and earlier death. Social isolation is very hard to take, even by very well adjusted and highly trained people, such as astronauts and cosmonauts, who know what they are in for. Valery Polyakov, the Russian cosmonaut who in 1994-95 set the record for the longest time in space (14 months), said afterwards: "It's a real effort to be away from everything. I mean, you are really isolated. They talk about the French Foreign Legion. Man, this is really…you're in the Sahara Desert, and there's just no way around it."

Numerous studies have shown that people who have a heart attack and are unmarried or lack emotional support are three times more likely to have a relapse than those who are not isolated in this way. And they die much sooner. John Cacioppo at the University of Chicago sees isolation as a health risk at any age, comparable to smoking and obesity. He and his group studied 2,632 undergraduate students. They found that even in a crowd there were some who found it difficult to make connections. They felt lonely even though they were not alone, and they had higher cortisol levels in the morning and throughout the day. "Lonely people view the world as a more threatening place," he commented. These observations emphasize the difference between "being alone" and "feeling lonely."

• Reach Out and Touch Somebody

The value of touching and hugging as part of social support therapy should not be underestimated. I ask people: "Do you touch with the fingers or the whole hand?" It makes a lot of difference to the soothing effectiveness of the touch. In Mediterranean and Latin American cultures, and in the days when we did not worry about sexual harassment, touching, patting someone's back or knee, and walking arm in arm were perfectly normal—tacit indicators of social support. Touch has important physiological benefits in its own right. Research among elderly populations at the University of Miami School of Medicine found those who are touched become more social, develop healthier habits, and get sick less often. People in loving relationships and happy marriages live longer. As long as you are able to, carry on making love. And hug often. There is nothing like a warm hug to make you feel good. Its healing power is very real. What's more, you can keep hugging long after sex fades.

• Get a Pet

Preferably, get a pet you can hug or stroke, like a cat or dog, or at least one you can talk to, like a canary or budgerigar. People who own dogs live longer. This may be true for cat-owners and those who keep other pets. Dogs show their unconditional affection by wagging their tail or licking you, and they instinctively know when you need comforting. They have an important added advantage. They make you take a walk at least once a day. That, in itself, is invaluable.

If you do not want to own a pet, how about starting a dog-walking service for neighbors? You do not walk too well? You can do it at your own pace, on flat terrain. You may make some pocket money on the side and expand your social network as you improve your health. Many more people will stop to pat your dog and talk to you than when you are walking alone. If you do not want an animal pet, talking to your plants is said to have similar soothing, stress-reducing effects.

• If You Must Worry, Save It for Later

Put off worrying by exercising, going for a walk, playing tennis, or enjoying a round of golf. Or go to a movie, a play, a concert, or an art gallery. Look for light, pleasant, amusing subjects. These activities give you a "time out" from stress. Invite some friends or neighbors for a tea party. Perhaps you may even be able to train yourself not to worry about things you can do nothing about.

Learning to Live with Change

There are many things you can do to reduce anxiety, and in the process you should also reduce your stress hormones. Just remember: it may not happen overnight. It took some time to get to the state you are in now. You may be anxious once in a while, or all the time. Try some of the approaches outlined above and see what works best for you.

Accept that life is full of problems and that you can't solve them all. Those who enjoy long, healthy lives have learned to accept change. Charles Darwin said, "It is not the strongest species that survive, nor the most intelligent, but the ones most responsive to change." People who accept change and respond to it do not get into a stew over frustrations they can do nothing about. There are many small steps you can take to manage your feelings of stress before they get out of control. The Chinese have a saying that a journey of a hundred miles begins with the first step. Just remember that stress is *feeling* out of control, not *being* out of control. Take action. Your life is at stake.

9

Managing What You Eat

○ ○

Sir, after examining my cholesterol profile, my doctor has told me that I should avoid eating cheese, butter, cream, eggs, liver, and many other fatty and cholesterol-rich foods. Now I am told that I should not eat pasta, rice, bread, or sugar. For heaven's sake, someone please tell me what I am allowed to eat, before all this stress causes me to have a heart attack.

—*John G. Francis, Letter to the editor,* The Times of London
(19 July 2002)

Living in space presents its own special problems. First of all, the amount of room in a spacecraft is extremely limited, so most of the astronauts' food has to be freeze dried to reduce its bulk. It is reconstituted when needed by adding water. Even as simple a task as cleaning your teeth is different in space. Imagine what it would be like flying around in conditions of near-zero gravity if everyone spat out their toothpaste in the mornings.

That is why space toothpaste is edible. It comes in many flavors—strawberry, banana, mint, and so on—and is meant to be swallowed. Another difference involves ice cream, one of the top two favorite desserts among astronauts (the other being crackerjacks). Too bulky to be loaded aboard in the normal state, space ice cream comes as granules. When popped into the mouth, these granules literally melt, taking on the flavor and texture of ice cream on Earth.

Apart from coping with the almost complete absence of gravity, astronauts have basically the same dietary requirements as those they leave behind on Earth, with some small but vital differences. Research is showing that being in space can impose special demands on the astronauts' diet. What they eat can, in fact, protect them from the damaging effects of space radiation and the oxidative damage of excessive stress. The amount of salt they eat may either protect their blood pressure responding system or, if there is too much, increase bone loss. It is believed that the maintenance of muscle mass depends on the amount and type of protein consumed and the time it is eaten relative to exercise.

Lose Fat with Gravity

Deprived of the daily challenge of gravity, the metabolism of astronauts in space is changed, with fat accumulating to replace lost muscle. The reduced motility and absorption of the gut alters the basic nutritive value of the foods they eat. We know that calcium, for instance, is not absorbed and glucose is not taken up by muscle as efficiently as they are in Earth's gravity. The sense of taste is altered. Food becomes bland and thirst is reduced, interfering with what astronauts may choose to eat or drink. Though a comprehensive study on nutrition and metabolism is very difficult to carry out in space and has not been done, much has been learned from studies in bed-rest volunteers. To make this information relevant to the general public this type of study should be done as well in others who are generally not very active, including children and the elderly.

However, fifty years ago it became possible to study the influence of gravity on metabolism more systematically. Milt Smith and Nello Pace built a centrifuge at the University of California, Davis, to house and expose animals, including chickens, mice, and rabbits, to hypergravity. They wanted to find out how living in gravity that was two or three times that of Earth's changed metabolism of living creatures. What they discovered, among other things, was a dramatic reduction of body fat. The animals ate the same amount of food except for the first few days, when they seemed to lose their appetites. Chickens, which normally had 33% body fat, ended up with only 3% fat after living for a few weeks at 3 G. Rabbits showed much the same change. Their level of activity was also reduced.

When the urine of these 3-G animals was injected into other rabbits living at 1 G, the body fat of the 1-G animals also decreased. Smith and his team were unable to pinpoint what had caused this totally unexpected result.

More recently, Chuck Fuller, a former student of Smith's, used the same centrifuge at UC Davis to follow up on these early observations. Fuller confirmed that mice living at 2G lost their appetites for the first few days. But six to eight weeks after adapting to the new gravity level, they were eating 22% more food. Their level of activity had picked up too, though it was still 40% lower than that of their litter mates living at 1 G. Despite this increased food consumption and lower activity, their body fat was almost half that of mice at 1 G. Later studies showed that the higher the G, the greater the fat loss.

This suggests that as you increase gravity, there is a metabolic shift toward a leaner state.

Imagine if you could harness the power of gravity to lose body fat by just spinning on a centrifuge. This may be a dream at present, but it is not an impossible one for the near future.

The Balanced Diet: For Some, a Once-in-a-Lifetime Experience

The first voluntary act performed by a newborn baby, after taking a good deep breath or two and announcing its arrival among us with a yell, is to look for food. For humans, as well as for other mammals, mother's milk provides the ideal combination of vitamins, minerals, proteins, and other nourishment needed for a baby to thrive.

For some, however, the period before being weaned may be the last time in their lives that they enjoy the full benefit of a balanced diet. In later life, particularly in the more prosperous countries, there are too many opportunities to eat foods that appeal to the taste buds but can, in excess, be disastrous for the rest of the body.

Surrounded by so many choices as we are in the USA, managing what you eat becomes essential. Knowing and understanding the values of foods can make the difference between damage and protection or healing.

No Bagels or Salty Snacks for the Cavemen

Our cavemen ancestors managed to survive without orange juice, bagels, and coffee for breakfast. And if they did not live as long as some of us do today, it was not because of their diet. They knew nothing of preservatives and insecticides, hormone-treated beef and chicken, salty snacks, or refined sugar.

Obesity and heart disease, so far as we know, were not common problems in the last Ice Age. People ate what they could find. In times of plenty they gorged; in times of scarcity they went without. Their staples were mostly raw fruit, nuts, vegetables, and roots. Meat or fish provided the occasional feast.

Reading the Labels

When my husband was diagnosed with Type-2 diabetes some years ago, I took to reading food labels with care. What a revelation! Previously I had taken just a swift glance at the saturated fat or sodium content listed on the label.

Most manufacturers have made great strides towards preparing healthier foods, and labeling laws have made the information listed more comprehensive and easier to read. But the main aim of food advertising, and this includes what goes on the label, is to make the contents of packets or cans more appealing. Unfortunately, it is we, the customers, who do not read labels carefully. Because something is labeled *diet* or *fat-free* does not mean it satisfies our specific health needs.

Hooked on Sugar

In her book, *The Origin Diet,* Elizabeth Somer, a registered dietitian, calculates that today we eat the equivalent of about twenty teaspoonfuls of refined sugar daily, an amount whose equivalent in fruit and honey our prehistoric ancestors probably consumed in a whole year. She bases this estimate on observations from anthropological remains that show essentially little tooth decay. I would say Somer's estimate of today's daily sugar intake is well on the conservative side.

A very health-conscious mother at our club swimming pool was offering her children, aged three and five, a small carton of fruit juice and a fruit roll for lunch. She could have realized that the juice contained 15–22 g of sugar and the roll 10–20 g, making a total for each child of 25–42 g. That's 6¾–11½ teaspoonfuls of sugar in a single meal!

What caught my attention was when I heard her tell them she was withholding the candy until later, because she did not want them to have too much sugar! Some schools in Virginia, I am told, offer young children a breakfast of fruit juice, chocolate milk, and a honey bun. The total nutritional element in such a meal is not exactly stellar, while the total sugar content alone is 81 g—equivalent to twenty-two teaspoonfuls of sugar. Please measure out that amount and take a good look at the heap. Now imagine eating it, a spoonful at a time, not to mention all the starch and fat in the bun. This is what some of us feed our children, thinking it a wholesome breakfast. This is unconscionable. It both creates and panders to a sweet tooth that will cause health problems throughout their lives.

The Enemies of Healthy Eating

Whether it happens at sixty-five or at eighty-five, we eventually face impediments in the path of our ability to eat well. Food can taste different from the way it used to, and appetites can diminish. There may not be sufficient resources to buy fresh food, or an older person may no longer be able to drive to the store. People at any age left on their own no longer have the motivation to cook a meal for one; others lack the know-how or do not manage what they eat properly by planning ahead. When they get hungry they are too impatient to wait for a meal to cook, so they eat whatever happens to be around. All of these factors work against healthy eating.

Then there are conflicting messages about what we should and should not eat. If you have high cholesterol, your doctor will tell you to "banish fats from your diet." If you have high blood pressure, "eliminate salt" is the advice. On the other hand, TV and magazines bombard us with highly professional advertisements for foods that often have high levels of fat and salt.

Pictures of your favorite sports stars imply that their achievements are due to eating a particular cereal. The poster of an anorexic-looking model biting into some tantalizing snack is meant to make you run to the store so that you can look like her. Fast-food chains add yet another layer of cheese, burger, or mayonnaise. The message is clear: keep putting tasty, high-calorie, low-nutrient junk food into your mouth. We have learned from space that inactivity is not good for you. However, coupled with unhealthy eating habits, it can be disastrous.

The 'Obesity Epidemic'

Have you ever wondered why you do not see too many obese people over eighty? The reason is quite simple: not many of them reach that age. Obesity puts people at risk from several life-shortening illnesses, including high blood pressure, blocked blood vessels due to cholesterol deposits, gallstones, diabetes, colon cancer, and arthritic degeneration of the joints.

And it is not only the elderly who need to be concerned. In a dietary environment that is dominated by fast foods, the current "obesity epidemic" is especially noticeable among children. It is not helped by a low level of physical activity and by a diet dominated by fast foods. In 1970, 5% of American teenagers and 7% of six to eleven-year-olds were considered overweight. By 1999, these numbers had grown to 14% for teenagers and 13% for the younger group. Among adults, a 2003 survey classified 44 million Americans as obese and another 68 million as overweight. That totals about 40% of the U.S. population. It is a shocking number!

Are You Overweight?

A figure known as the Body Mass Index (BMI) is used to decide whether or not an individual is carrying too much weight. It is calculated by applying the formula W/H2—the weight in kilograms divided by the square of the height in meters. (To turn kilograms into pounds, multiply by 2.2, and to turn meters into inches, multiply by 39.4.) Thus, a man measuring 1.8 m (5 ft 11 in) and weighing 80 kg (176 lb) will have a BMI of 24.7.

The desirable BMI for men is 21.9 to 22.4, and for women it is 21.3 to 22.1. A BMI between 25 and 30 is considered overweight and anything above 30 is defined as obese. Muscular athletes with low-body fat are the exception to these definitions, for they can have a high BMI without being obese. BMI charts can be found on the Internet health site www.consumer.gov/weight-loss/bmi.htm.

The Bigger the Plate, the Bigger the Threat

Marion Nestle at New York University lambasted the eating habits of the U.S. public in her book, *Food Politics*. In explaining how the food industry and the food interest lobbies spend $10 billion a year to promote overeating, she points out how larger plates and more generous portions at restaurants showed up in the late 1970s—the same time obesity was making its mark. She also draws attention to the fact that bigger bagels and muffins have more sugar and fat to make them "taste good." And she says that the public is encouraged to buy potato chips rather than potatoes, because "that is where the profit is."

I particularly support her views on cereals. In the early 1980s, I remember taking Galya, a visiting colleague from the Soviet Union, to a supermarket and then watching her jaw drop at the multitude of cereals on display. "Why do you need so many different kinds?" she asked. I had never thought how overwhelming such a variety of choices were, and I felt embarrassed at how lucky we were in our free society to have so much choice. But equally embarrassing was the fact that most cereals on the supermarket shelves were loaded with sugar. There are very few cereals on the supermarket shelves that can be eaten by diabetics and those who are serious about cutting down their sugar intake.

Basic corn flakes, oatmeal, and shredded wheat usually contain about 1–2 grams of sugar per serving (1 cup). Anything over that is too much, for two reasons. First, cereal is only one of many foods containing sugar that will be eaten during the day, so the total daily sugar will mount up. Secondly, we should avoid spikes in the level of sugar in the blood.

A cup of plain corn flakes, in addition to the added sugar that enters the blood directly, provides 21 g of other carbohydrates that promptly get converted into sugar. If you add half a cup of skimmed milk (6 g sugar), you end up with a total of 8 g of sugar and 21 g of other carbohydrates—a sizeable and damaging sugar jolt. In many breakfast cereals, as much as half the calories can come from the added sugar alone.

Processed and packaged foods often contain more sugar, salt, and saturated fats than is good for health. They are added because they improve the flavor.

How to Read Labels

The National Academy of Sciences advises that every day you should eat at least three servings of whole grain foods, such as bread, cereals, rice, or pasta. But the labeling on grains can be misleading. *Multigrain, stone ground,* and *whole grain* are often just terms the manufacturer uses to mislead you into thinking that the product contains all the fiber you believe you are getting. Unless the label shows *whole wheat* or *whole oat* listed first in the ingredients, you may be getting duped. The higher their fiber content, the better. A dark, healthy-looking loaf of bread may be that way because of caramel or molasses added for color rather than bran. The moral: *read your labels.*

Read the whole label, not just part of it, including serving size, number of calories per serving size, fat, protein, and carbohydrate content, and any special claims made. Ingredients are listed in descending order by weight. Check the percentage of your recommended daily intake of minerals, vitamins, fiber, and other nutrients you are getting in a single serving. Here are two examples of labels, the one on the left for a shredded wheat whole grain cereal without added milk, the one on the right for a popular "fat free" plain yogurt.

Food Cravings

You probably have moments when your body craves salt, but the answer does not have to be salty pretzels or potato chips. A few salted nuts, such as peanuts or almonds, are a healthier option. Or you may feel tired or cold and need some fuel, so you reach for a comforting glazed doughnut. You will be getting a lot of extra fat and carbohydrate with your sugar fix. A cup of hot cocoa without sugar should satisfy your craving.

If you are healthy and active, your body will let you know what you need. Listen to it. Understand labels. Use common sense to make smart choices. Know what you are eating and what you need to eat.

Nutrition Facts

	Shredded Wheat		Fat-Free Yogurt	
	Amount per Serving	% Daily Values	Amount per Serving	% Daily Values
Total Fat	1g	0%	0g	0%
Saturated Fat	0g	0%	0g	0%
Cholesterol	0mg	0%	5mg	2%
Sodium	130mg	5%	190mg	8%
Potassium	120mg	3%	590mg	8%
Total Carb.	28g	9%	19g	6%
Dietary Fiber	4g	16%	0g	0%
Sugars	2g		17g	
Protein	4g	8%	12g	24%
Vitamin A		0%		0%
Vitamin C		0%		0%
Calcium		0%		40%
Iron		6%		0%
Serving size	35 g (about 1 cup)		8 oz/227 g (1 cup)	
Calories per serving	120		130	
Calories from fat	0		0	

The benefits of the shredded wheat, as shown by the label above, lie in its high fiber content (16% of your daily requirement) and, for a cereal, its very low sugar content (2 g, or about half a teaspoon, per serving). Its carbohydrate content provides 9% of your daily intake in a form that is absorbed more slowly than sugars, thereby minimizing spikes in your blood sugar level. By contrast, although the yogurt provides almost half of your daily calcium requirement and a fair amount of protein, its carbohydrate is almost all in the form of sugar.

Three Inventions That Lure Us into Dodging Gravity

Inactivity is a way of dodging gravity. Being active implies moving about, but any movement is virtually useless unless we are working against the force of gravity or using resistance against a similar force. Not so long ago, the pioneers going West or setting up farms had to dig and plow, plant and harvest, milk the cows, and chase after strays. They did not know what it was to lead an inactive life. How do our lifestyles compare?

Perhaps the most significant inventions contributing to our present inactive state are the internal combustion engine, the television, and the microchip. There is something incongruous about jumping into a car to go to the supermarket across the street and then spending thirty minutes on a treadmill to stay "fit." The microchip is now found in every home and office. It has an impact on our lives through television, videos, computers, banking systems, and mobile phones.

Its impact on our children and grandchildren is even greater. Soon people will not even need to go to the doctor, because diagnosis and treatment will be done through telemedicine. Groceries can already be ordered and delivered, with meals prepackaged and ready to heat up, all from the comfort of your chair or bed. In theory, there could be no need to get up at all—except perhaps to exercise! This is true for the older person, and especially for those who live alone.

The Perils of Dodging Gravity

Predicting the future is an inexact science. But if present trends continue and inactivity, spurred by labor-saving inventions, becomes more and more prevalent, the outlook for our health is far from cheerful. The human frame, with all its nerves, bones, muscles, and blood vessels, evolved under the influence of one of the most powerful forces in the universe—gravity. As long as we plan to live on Earth in reasonably good health, it is essential to be aware of that force and to exploit its benefits by staying active.

The consequences to the body when gravity is removed or drastically reduced can be seen in "fast forward" when astronauts voyage into space or volunteers spend several weeks in continuous bed rest. Those who choose inactivity will find that their muscles and bones grow weaker because the demands made on them by gravity are reduced. Lying down for much of the day, instead of walking around or simply standing upright, means that the heart, relieved of its task of pumping blood to the head, will become weaker too.

As if these drawbacks were not enough, "couch potatoes" will inevitably become fatter unless they make an effort to cut down on the amount they eat.

Somebody who is lying down burns up only about one calorie a minute. Standing up results in an energy expenditure a shade under two calories a minute, or 119 calories per hour for a 165-lb man over sixty years of age, and 97 calories per hour for a 132-lb woman. This means we burn twice as many calories when we stand as when we are lying down.

If you want to neither gain weight nor lose it, the amount of food consumed needs to be in balance, calorie for calorie, with the amount of activity taken. The nature of the food has a bearing on this. One gram of fat contains nine calories, whereas 1 g of protein or carbohydrate provides four calories. An elderly person lying in bed or who is less active than before needs fewer calories than when he or she was physically active.

How Much Water Do We Need?

The body uses water to transport its nutrients and waste materials, and every cell depends on water for its survival. For these reasons, the amount of water in the body is very tightly regulated. Dehydration brings constipation, skin dryness, faintness, exhaustion, and sometimes nausea. The body may overheat and the risk of kidney stones increases. And the proportion of water in the body decreases with age. That is why it is important to drink more water as we get older.

In men, water accounts for about 60% of the bodyweight until around age forty, but it comes down to just over 50% by the age of eighty or ninety. In women it starts decreasing much earlier, at eighteen, and by age sixty it falls as low as 46%. This is partly because women have more body fat, and gain still more with age, for fat cells contain far less water than lean muscle cells.

The initial rapid loss of weight achieved by many diets, and sometimes as a side effect of disease or aging, is usually due to loss of water. The body's water supply comes not just from drinking but also from food and as a by-product in the process of burning fuel to generate energy. Water is lost in sweat, urine, feces, and water vapor breathed out.

To cover essential water needs, adults of average size and build should take in four to six cups of water a day if they are inactive, and eight cups or more if they are active. This does not all have to come from water that is drunk. Water in the food you eat should always be considered in the total water requirement. Soup, hot drinks, gelatin desserts, fresh fruit, and salads all provide a considerable proportion of the daily requirement, though frequently they are not counted in the water intake. Those who have difficulty drinking a lot of water because they are not thirsty or do not enjoy the taste should make sure they get plenty of food items with a high water content.

Dehydration reduces blood volume. Less blood circulating means less oxygen being carried around the body, and this reduces aerobic capacity during exercise or strenuous activity. Drinking a 12-oz glass of water (355ml) one hour before exercising can extend endurance and strength. Frederick Stare, who recently died at ninety-one, founded the department of nutrition at Harvard in 1942. He was a strong supporter of drinking water "to protect the joints from stiffness, aid digestion, and keep wrinkles at bay." Dr Stare's two watchwords for remaining healthy were "prudence and moderation."

The Toilet Dilemma in Space

Astronauts in space as well as inactive people and the elderly here on Earth have a lower blood volume, are dehydrated, and also tend to be less thirsty. Astronauts put out less urine because they drink even less than the other two groups. This may not be simply a matter of feeling less thirsty—it may also be because using the space toilet takes more time and is more complicated than here on Earth. Yes, there is a toilet on the Shuttle and the International Space Station, but it is not simple to use, because you must be well secured to the seat to avoid floating away. Astronauts tend not to use the toilet in the spacecraft as often as they might.

Astronaut and physician Rhea Seddon and her scientist colleagues noted that astronauts intentionally dehydrated themselves by restricting what they drank before launch, to avoid lying in wet diapers in their space suits during the countdown to lift-off. Some have also done so in the belief that it may reduce the nausea that can accompany the first few days in space. It is not known to what extent decreased fluid consumption among the elderly is aggravated by a wish to avoid using a toilet—possibly because they might have to call on someone for help.

How Much Food Is Enough?

The National Research Council developed a formula to calculate energy expenditure, and hence caloric needs, taking into account age, gender, weight, and level of activity. According to this formula, 1,432 calories per day would meet the daily dietary needs of an inactive 70-kg (154-lb) man over sixty spending most of his time in bed. An inactive 70-kg thirty to sixty-year-old man would need 1,691 calories per day. A 55-kg (121-lb) inactive woman over sixty would need no more than 1,174 calories a day, whereas one between thirty to sixty years old would need 1,308 calories. These caloric needs are increased by an activity factor if they were walking about and carrying out their normal daily activities. The over-sixty men and women would need 2,291 and 1,878 calories per day, respectively.

They would need still more calories if they took up exercise, depending on its intensity and duration. When someone resumes an active life after more than thirty days in bed, it takes three to six weeks for the metabolic rate (the rate at which calories are burned) to return to normal. This is why people with a sedentary lifestyle who start exercising to lose weight often become discouraged when no immediate results are seen.

Energy Needs of Men and Women Over 60

	Body Weight kg	Body Weight lb	Calories Required per Day Inactive	Calories Required per Day Active
MEN	65	143	1,365	2,184
	70	154	1,432	2,291
	75	165	1,500	2,400
	80	176	1,566	2,506
	85	187	1,635	2,616
WOMEN	50	110	1,121	1,794
	55	121	1,174	1,878
	60	132	1,226	1,962
	70	154	1,331	2,130
	75	165	1,384	2,214

Inactive means staying in bed without using muscles
for any physical activity.
Active means being up and going about one's daily activities.
Source: Data in *National Research Council Recommended Dietary
Allowances*, 10th ed. (Washington, D.C.: National Academy Press, 1989).

Paradoxically, one way to lose weight is to lie in bed continuously. This is confirmed by what happens to healthy volunteers participating in bed-rest studies or to patients confined to bed at home or in hospital. The weight loss is initially due to greater loss of water by diuresis, the excessive discharge of urine. The hormones that regulate water sense an increased fluid volume in the upper body when somebody is lying down. They are mobilized to reduce this volume by increasing urine output and reducing thirst.

Another factor contributing to a loss of weight is that water is one of the by-products of burning calories to provide the body's energy. But lying in bed means that less energy is needed and fewer calories are burned. Appetite and thirst are reduced, but most importantly there is a shift in the muscle cells from lean muscle to fat. Muscles use protein as fuel when they contract. Unused, they quickly shrink, and the food that is taken in and not burned is stored as fat. Fat weighs less than muscle, so you may believe you are losing weight when in fact you are getting fatter!

The Case for Fats

Fat is among the chief nutritional components of food. It is that greasy solid or semi-solid compound that does not dissolve in water. We get our fat by eating meats, milk, cream, cheese, oils, fish oils, and nuts. It is also added to processed foods, especially snacks, to enhance flavor.

Fats provide more than twice as much energy per gram (9 calories) as carbohydrates or proteins (4 calories in each case). They are the source of the important essential fatty acids needed in the production and storage of energy and in stabilizing blood sugar. Fats also provide the insulation and cushioning needed by the skin, bones, and internal organs. And they carry and store certain vitamins such as A, D, E or K. Some fats form part of the outer membrane of every cell in the body. Others, such as cholesterol, are essential for the production of sex hormones and adrenal hormones.

But although there is no question that we need fats in our diet, the exact daily requirement has not been established beyond argument. Fats make up about 40–50% of the total calories in the average diet in the USA, and many nutritionists consider this amount excessive. In Mediterranean countries, where the diet is considered very healthy, the amount of fat eaten is half of that in the USA. The astronauts' diet now provides 30–35% of their total dietary calories in the form of fats.

Measuring Body Fat

There are several methods of measuring body fat, which can be found at some health clubs, doctors' offices, or medical centers. None are very accurate, so the results should be taken only as a general guide. Fat shows up very nicely on a MRI (Magnetic Resonance Imaging) of leg muscles. The less sophisticated skin-fold test relies on pinching the skin together at three to seven sites of the body, such as the back of the arm, the abdomen, inner thigh, and "love handles" around the waist.

A skinfold caliper is usually a simple two-pronged plastic or metal compass-like device that gives you a reading of the thickness of each fold. It is one of the better methods when done by a well-trained person or by the same person each time. At twenty, an active young man's body is about 18% fat and a woman's is between 14% and 25%. An average obese man of that age has more than 25% fat, and an obese woman more than 35%. By the age of sixty, the average fit man's body fat will have more than doubled to 38%, while the woman's will have increased to 44%.

Body builders, weightlifters, and athletes who train with weights may suffer disastrous consequences if they stop suddenly because of injury or at the end of a career. Beautiful muscles that took so much effort to build will very quickly be replaced by fat. It takes just as much care and determination as it did during their years of training for human beings that were once highly active to adjust to a lower level of activity. They need to reduce their activity, food intake, and weight very gradually if they want to come down to a muscle mass that they can maintain in their new non-competitive lifestyle.

Good and Bad Fats

As far as the human body is concerned, not all fats are created equal. Understanding their advantages and disadvantages is at the root of good fat management. In general, saturated fats are bad, unsaturated fats are good, and essential fatty acids are best.

The Benefits of Eating Oily Fish

Essential fatty acids are the "good" fats that are needed by the body for health and growth. They are called essential because they cannot be made by the body but can only be obtained from what we eat. These fats are found in oily fish such as salmon, mackerel, and sardines. They contain omega-3 and omega-6 fatty acids, which are very effective in reducing the risk of heart disease and protecting the brain from inflammation when insulin is excessive.

Unsaturated fats, as distinct from the harmful saturated fats, are usually liquid. They include plant oils such as corn oil, cottonseed oil, olive oil, and canola oil (made from a kind of rapeseed). Olive oil and canola oil have beneficial effects in lowering excessive cholesterol. Both oils contain high amounts of alpha-linolenic acid, which is rich in omega-3 and omega-6 and are powerful anti-inflammatory agents.

Serge Reynaud at the University of Lyons, France, reported in 1994 the results of a study in 600 individuals who had suffered a coronary heart attack. Half of them were given a diet rich in alpha-linolenic acid, while the other half were put on the low-fat diet that is usually prescribed for heart patients. After four years,

70% fewer deaths and recurrences of heart attacks were recorded among the first group.

Nuts are a good source of monounsaturated or polyunsaturated fat, which lowers excessive cholesterol. Some seeds such as flax are very rich in linolenic acid. Walnuts are the only nut with a high amount of alpha-linolenic acid, the only type of omega-3 fat found in plants, and they are rich in vitamin E as well. Other nuts, such as almonds, peanuts, pistachios, and pecans, are also rich in vitamin E. Unfortunately, their high fat content—160–200 calories per ounce—has subdued our love for nuts. About 80% of their calories come from fat. And who stops after eating only one ounce.

Fats That Harm

The relationship between a high-fat diet and diseases such as blocked blood vessels, heart attacks, strokes, gallstones, and colon cancer has received a great deal of attention. The worst offenders in this respect are "saturated fats," which are usually solid at room temperature. They include animal fats; dairy products, such as butter, cream, and cheese; meat; chocolate; and coconut. The body also makes its own saturated fats.

A diet low in saturated fats, which is highly advisable for anybody at risk of a stroke or heart attack, means cutting down on eggs, whole milk, cream, butter, and coconut oil, as well as hydrogenated fats, such as margarine or cooking fats, and fatty meats, especially beef. This helps to keep blood cholesterol within its desirable range of 100–199 mg per 100 ml of blood. Anything above that amount can clog up arteries and cause heart attacks and stroke.

Trans-fatty acids are potentially harmful unsaturated fats produced when a liquid vegetable oil is solidified by the process of hydrogenation. They are considered a health risk because they raise cholesterol. For this reason they will soon be listed on food labels.

We hear much about "good" and "bad" cholesterol. These terms actually refer to the high-density (HDL) and low density lipoproteins in our blood, which have the capacity to bind fats and clear them from the bloodstream. As its name implies, HDL has a higher number of fat-binding sites and is more effective in clearing up cholesterol from the blood. If you have a medical check-up, the normal range for HDL is 35–150 mg per 100 ml of blood, and for LDL it is 0–129 mg per 100 ml. Lower HDL or higher LDL would be a cause for concern.

The best way to ensure that there is a high HDL level in the blood is to exercise vigorously. An increase in HDLs, or "good" cholesterol, has been shown to lower the risk of atherosclerosis—the plaque that blocks blood vessels. Obese people, diabetics, and those who are physically inactive, on the other hand, have high levels of LDL in the blood, which increases their risk of suffering a stroke.

Fats That Can Trigger Alzheimer's Disease

Recently, a link was established between the amount of fat in the diet and Alzheimer's disease. Robert Friedland at Case Western Reserve University School of Medicine, in Cleveland, Ohio, analyzed decades of eating patterns in 304 elderly men and women, 72 of whom had Alzheimer's. They found that people with the susceptibility gene for Alzheimer's (Apo-E4) who had eaten high saturated-fat diets between age twenty and sixty had an eight times greater incidence of the disease than those who had the gene but had lived on a low-fat diet.

The Apo-E4 gene also increases susceptibility to cardiovascular disease. High-saturated-fat diets when we are twenty to forty can come back to haunt us in our later years if we have a predisposition towards either of these diseases. About 40 to 44% of the population carry the Apo-E4 gene.

Protein in the Diet

Bones, cartilage, muscles, hormones, and the immune system are made up mainly of protein. It is crucial for growth and development, because it provides support for the body's cells and builds and repairs muscles and other body tissue. Proteins are built from amino acids, and though many of these can be made in the body, there are nine that we can only obtain from the food we eat. They are found in meat, poultry, fish, dairy products, soy beans, nuts, fruit, and vegetables.

Muscles contain about a quarter of all the protein in the body. Another 25% of protein is found throughout the abdominal organs, in the immune system, and in the blood. The other 50% of proteins make up the collagen and elastin that form the bulk of support structures in the body—the bones, skin, joints, and tendons.

Elastin and collagen turn over, that is, they break down and are rebuilt, very slowly, over years. But muscle, organ, and blood proteins turn over within a few days. Continuous protein turnover requires a lot of energy, which can come only from the food we eat. We make and break down about 300 g of protein every day. Unused protein is not stored but eliminated from the body. This is in contrast to carbohydrates, which are stored as glycogen in the liver and muscles, and as fat in fatty tissues.

A Reverse Order Breakfast?

Dermatologist Nicolas Perricone in his book, *The Perricone Prescription*, recommends: "Eat your protein first at every meal." Protein is slowly digested, so it will delay and smooth out the increase in blood sugar from the carbohydrate on your plate. This is an interesting and useful technique. According to this approach, you should have your eggs and bacon before your cereals, and your chicken or fish before your rice at dinner.

If the body does not get enough fat and carbohydrates, it uses protein for energy. In cases of malnutrition, anorexia, or an inadequate supply of amino acids in the diet, the amount of protein made is reduced. The result is a thin, frail body. Older people can suffer protein loss through not eating enough, not having a balanced diet, being inactive, or being under stress.

Eventually, the structural proteins in collagen and elastin break down, and the immune system collapses because immune proteins are not made in the blood. If 30 to 40% of total body protein is lost, as happens in extreme anorexia, the usual result is death

Carbohydrates, the 'Energy' Foods

There are three kinds of carbohydrates: sugars, starches, and cellulose; the first two are the principal sources of energy for the body. The sugars, known as simple carbohydrates, are found naturally in all sugars, honey, milk, and fruit. They are added to many foods and soft drinks. Starches, the so-called complex carbohydrates, are found in potatoes, rice, bread, pasta, and various kinds of peas and beans. Cellulose is fiber that comes from the plants we eat. It is not digestible but plays an important role in exercising the digestive system by providing roughage.

Sugars and refined processed starches, such as white flour, increase blood sugar very quickly, causing spikes. This sets up a vicious cycle. First, insulin increases to reduce this high blood-sugar level. Then blood sugar drops, making you hungry, so you eat more. Your blood sugar then soars again, and the cycle continues. Inevitably you put on more weight, because the sugar spikes are making you eat more than you need. To manage your carbohydrates, it is very important to avoid sugar spikes—or at the very least to smooth them out.

Complex carbohydrates, on the other hand, which are found in whole grain foods such as brown rice, have a high fiber content, so they increase blood sugar more slowly, providing a steady supply over a longer period.

All sugars and starches, once digested, are converted into the simplest sugar, glucose. Transported in the blood, glucose is burned as fuel to provide energy or is stored for future use. The hormone insulin, secreted by the pancreas, facilitates the transport of any unused glucose into the liver and muscle cells, where it is stored as glycogen. If insufficient carbohydrate is eaten, other sources of energy, such as fat or protein, can be used as fuel for most parts of the body, but glucose is the only source of energy for the brain.

The Danger in Crash Diets

If carbohydrates are restricted excessively, as in some weight-loss "crash" diets, the body starts drawing on its glycogen "bank." Depending on how low the amount of carbohydrate in the diet is, all the glycogen stored in the liver can be used up in as little as three days. This can be the beginning of the process termed "starvation," when the body turns to its protein and fat stores for energy. The early and rapid weight loss experienced with most low-carbohydrate diets comes from the loss of water that was stored with the glycogen. The weight will be gained back as soon as the dieter starts eating carbohydrates again.

Nutritionists generally recommend that for people who are dieting, no less than 25% of the total calories consumed should come from carbohydrates. In the astronaut diet, as in the USA in general, it is closer to 50%. Today, no more than 5% of the carbohydrates the astronauts eat is sugar. They eat mostly complex carbohydrates—starches from grains and cereals, with their bran, that need to be digested and metabolized and therefore provide the desired slow-digesting, long-lasting source of glucose.

The Glycemic Index

A new school of thought now recommends that carbohydrates should be assessed on their glycemic index (GI)—a term taken from the Greek word *glykos* (sweet) and *heme* (blood). This is based on the effect various foods have on the blood-sugar level two to three hours after being eaten.

How Different Foods Affect Your Blood Sugar

Below, the glycemic index (GI) numbers for some common foods are shown. The GI ranks food items on a scale of 1–100, with 100 representing the highest possible level of glucose in the blood two to three hours after the food has been eaten. Ratings can vary with the method of food preparation or processing. The GI of fruit rises as it ripens. For instance, an under-ripe banana is 43, whereas it is 74 when it has ripened.

French Baguette	95	Whole Wheat Bread	69
Carrots	95	Croissant	67
Corn Flakes	82	Refined Sugar	65
Rice Krispies	82	Potatoes	65
Brown Rice, long grain	79	Honey	58–67
Bran Flakes, no raisins	74	Corn	55
Bananas, ripe	74	Bananas, under-ripe	43
Bagel	72	Soybeans	25

By choosing foods with a lower GI you can avoid unhealthy large surges in blood sugar after a meal.

Rebalancing the Diet

If you cut down on exercise and physical activity in general, you will tend to lose your appetite for protein, particularly for meat and fish. For this reason, it has been traditionally considered desirable to increase the amount of protein in the diet of inactive elderly people and to reduce their fat and carbohydrate intake. Whereas a normal diet would contain 15% protein, 50% carbohydrate, and 35% fat, the usual recommendation for sedentary or bedridden people are that the proportions be changed to 32% protein, 40% carbohydrate, and 28% fat.

The Astronaut's Diet

The loss of appetite for protein is also something that happens to astronauts in space, where food tends to taste blander. Their diet is designed to provide about 3,000 calories a day for a 75-kg (165-lb) man and about 2,160 calories for a 60-kg (132-lb) woman. This is the amount of calories they need on the ground, with their intense exercising regime, and the same amount is provided to them in space. Another 500 calories are added for times of even greater exertion, as when working outside the spacecraft.

In the early days of spaceflight, the diet contained a high proportion of sugary foods in order to provide instant energy. Today, the diet is made up of 15% protein, 35% fat, and 50% carbohydrate. To ensure that astronauts get all the amino acids they need, 60% of the protein comes from animal sources such as meat, chicken, fish, and cheese, against 40% from plant sources, such as nuts. Though the total amount of fat in the astronaut diet may seem high, these are mostly mono-unsaturated fats, such as olive oil, which has antioxidant properties and protects cells from damage.

The carbohydrates come from many sources, but as much as 95% is from complex carbohydrates, which have high fiber content and are relatively slow to turn into sugar in the body. They include bran, beans, and whole-grain products, to provide the roughage that enables the body to function properly.

Sample Menus for the International Space Station

	Day 1	Day 2	Day 3
Breakfast	Z Scrambled eggs/bacon Sausage, hash T Milk Z Juice, apple R Coffee/Tea/Cocoa	NF Cereal, cold T Yogurt, fruit T Juice, cranberry R Coffee/Tea/Cocoa	Z French toast Z Bacon, Canadian Z Margarine T Syrup Z Juice, orange R Coffee/Tea/Cocoa

Lunch	Z Chicken, oven fried
	T Macaroni and cheese
	T Corn, whole Kernel
	T Peaches
	NF Nuts, almonds
	TJ juice, pineapple-
	      Grapefruit
		T Soup, cream of
		      broccoli
		Z Beef patty
		FF Cheese slice
		Z Sandwich bun
		NF Pretzel
		NF Dried apples
		R Instant breakfast,
		      chocolate
			Z Cheese manicotti/
			      tomato sauce
			Z Bread, garlic
			Z Berry medley
			NF Cookies,
			      shortbread
			Z Lemonade
			T Pudding, vanilla

Dinner	Z Beef fajita
	T Rice, Spanish
	NF Tortilla chips
	T Picante sauce
	T Chile con queso
	T Tortilla
	Z Lemon bar
	R Apple cider
		Z Fish sautéed
		T Tartar sauce
		T Lemon Juice
		T Salad, pasta
		T Green beans
		Z Bread
		Z Margarine
		Z Angel food cake
		Z Strawberries
		R Drink, orange-
		      pineapple
			Z Turkey breast,
			      sliced
			Z Mashed sweet
			      potato
			T Asparagus tips
			Z Cornbread
			Z Margarine
			Z Pie, pumpkin
			R Drink, cherry

Key: Z   = Frozen
     R   = Rehydratable
    NF = Natural form
    T   = Thermostabilized
    F   = Fresh

Source: NASA

The Recommended Daily Allowance for fiber is 23% of total calorie intake. No more than 5% of the carbohydrates may come directly from sugar.

Who's for Spinach?

Within the guidelines set out to provide a balanced diet, the astronauts are given a fairly wide choice between individual food items, and all have their personal preferences. Spinach, it seems, is not high on the list. Before any mission into space, the astronauts spend a lot of time in simulations—rehearsals for the journey to come. I well recall being invited to take part in a simulation for the Space Life Science (SLS) 2 mission that flew in December 1993 and choosing the creamed spinach, one of my favorite dishes. The commander, John Blaha, the pilot, Rick Searfoss, and the rest of the crew looked at one another amused. Here was a person who actually liked spinach.

Bill Evans at the University of Arkansas argues that astronauts should get more protein. He carried out experiments to evaluate how much protein they and we need and what happens to it. He concludes that at least 20% of total calories in the diet should come from protein. More protein will be critical to reducing muscle loss on longer spaceflights.

On Earth, 20% of protein in the diet is acceptable, as long as it is consumed over the course of the day. For those who wish to build up muscle, Evans found that protein is most effective if consumed within thirty minutes of weight training exercise, when the muscles mop it up avidly. Taken a mere two hours after the end of exercising, the protein had no effect on muscle building, for the muscles did not take it up. Similarly, a cocktail of essential amino acids will increase protein synthesis most efficiently if it is consumed just before exercise.

Preventing Constipation

Constipation is a frequent complication of physical inactivity or prolonged bed rest. It is a hazard, too, for astronauts on a spaceflight. But steps are taken to prevent it by ensuring that the astronaut diet contains a good proportion of fiber. There are lessons in this for older people and for anybody else who might suffer from constipation.

In space, because the motility of the gut is reduced, it takes more time for food to transit through the gastrointestinal tract. This increases the potential for constipation, because more water is absorbed into the body the longer the stool remains in the intestines. Similar reduced gastrointestinal motility may occur in people who are confined to bed after surgery and in the less active elderly. Being up and about helps prevent these symptoms. Eating a diet rich in fiber from salads, vegetables, fruits, and bran, drinking plenty of water, and staying active is the best prescription to ward off constipation.

Missing Out on Nutrients

In space and in bed-rest, the gut becomes less efficient at absorbing nutrients from the bloodstream. A reduction in the amount of calcium absorbed has been documented both in astronauts during spaceflight and in healthy volunteers during bed-rest. This is of great concern, since it can aggravate the loss of calcium from bone that already occurs in both situations. And it is not just the absorption of nutrients that suffers. Reduced drug absorption was first suspected when drugs were found to be ineffective in treating space sickness and helping astronauts sleep.

Apart from a reduced absorption of calcium, it is not known to what extent the absorption of other nutrients, vitamins, and minerals is also reduced by inactivity in older people. I would predict, however, that this effect is widespread. Such diminished absorption would mean that older persons are not getting their minimum daily nutritional requirements.

Astronauts get vitamin supplements in space, whereas they do not need them here on Earth. Older folk, especially if they are less active, must take vitamins and mineral supplements. It would also benefit them to become more active and keep eating a healthy diet rich in fruit and vegetables.

The Highs and Lows of Blood Sugar

One of the hazards of an inactive life is a dramatic change for the worse in the way the body handles glucose. A healthy body keeps glucose in the blood at a level between 65 and 110 mg per 100 ml. If it drops below this level, we feel faint and tired and need to eat a high-energy food, such as orange juice or chocolate, to give the blood sugar a boost.

Some people suffer from hypoglycemia (low blood sugar) and have to snack throughout the day, taking their carbohydrate in small, frequent portions to maintain a steady level of glucose in the blood. A large slug of sugar triggers the release of insulin from the pancreas in order to get the excess glucose out of the blood and into the muscle cells. In some people, the insulin is so effective that glucose in the blood takes a nosedive, which in extreme cases can lead to a hypoglycemic coma.

At the other extreme are the diabetics, who suffer from hyperglycemia (high blood sugar). This condition, too, can lead to coma. Diabetes is a disorder in which the level of blood sugar is out of control. In Type-1 diabetes the pancreas cannot produce insulin at all. In Type-2 diabetes muscle does not take up glucose efficiently because it is less sensitive to insulin. To make matters worse, not enough insulin is produced by the pancreas to manage the abnormally high glucose levels.

Type-1 usually develops in childhood and requires the lifelong injection of insulin. Type-2 develops mostly in middle age. However, it is starting to affect younger people, and even teenagers, especially those who are overweight. Type-2 diabetes can usually be controlled by diet, activity, and pills.

If the blood-sugar level is not controlled, the consequences can be disastrous. Glucose attaches itself to the outer surfaces of body cells, causing them to stiffen and leak. This can lead to blindness, leaky blood vessels in the legs, poor circulation, reduced libido, impotence, heart disease, high blood pressure, kidney failure, and the inability of the immune system to heal wounds. In some cases, a limb may have to be amputated.

Nature's Warning Sign

In otherwise healthy people who are overweight and not as active as they might be, there is an intermediate condition known as the "pre-diabetic state." In this condition, glucose levels stay high because insulin is less effective in pushing glucose from the blood into the muscle cells. The pancreas, reacting to this continued high blood sugar, puts out more and more insulin. High levels of insulin can in themselves be damaging, causing inflammation. The "pre-diabetic" state is the body's warning sign, and the condition is reversible if it is diagnosed at an early stage and if the person concerned is prepared to cut down on sugar-rich foods and adopt a more active lifestyle. If uncontrolled, it will proceed to Type-2 diabetes, which is irreversible. Inactivity, then, in other words not using gravity effectively, is a major factor in the development of Type-2 diabetes.

Testing for Diabetes

Sometimes, pills that lower insulin resistance are helpful until the lifestyle adjustment has been made. If you are inactive, obese, crave sweets, or need to urinate often you could very well be in the pre-diabetic stage. Ask your doctor for an Oral Glucose Tolerance Test (OGTT). The test is taken after fasting for ten hours to diagnose the presence of diabetes. If your fasting blood glucose is between 75 and 110 mg per 100 ml and the level rises to between 140 and 190 mg within two hours of drinking the sugary drink that is part of the test, you are considered a "pre-diabetic." If your fasting sugar is greater than 126 mg and goes over 200 mg within two hours, you already have diabetes.

High blood glucose and excessive insulin levels after an OGTT have been measured in people confined to wheelchairs, in the victims of spinal cord injury, in healthy people during bed rest, and in others confined to bed for prolonged periods without any change in diet. Our research has shown that resistance to the action of insulin develops in all these inactive states. Insulin resistance is also seen in people who are obese and in elderly people and is attributed to a life of reduced activity and to a diet high in saturated fats.

By contrast, exceptionally active people use up glucose to obtain energy most efficiently. In an experiment in the 1960s, the super fit members of the Norwegian Ski Patrol showed only tiny increases in their blood-sugar and insulin levels after a standard OGTT.

More and more people these days are being diagnosed with diabetes, which can be a killer disease. Some 16.8 million Americans were diagnosed with Type-2 diabetes in 2003. The rate at which Type-2 diabetics are increasing has tripled in the last thirty years. It is more than coincidence that obesity in the general population has increased over the same period.

Oxygen, Free Radicals, and Antioxidants

This is a story of good news, bad news, and more good news. The good news is that we have lots of oxygen around us to breathe in order to stay alive. The bad news is that using oxygen to burn calories and generate energy leaves our body cells with some undesirable by-products: the high-energy molecules known as "free radicals."

Normal molecules have pairs of electrons attached to them and are relatively stable. But the electrons in free radical molecules are not paired, and this makes them unstable. To achieve stability, these "rogue" molecules commandeer electrons from other molecules, making them unstable in turn and setting up a chain reaction within the body. This can cause serious damage to cell membranes, to proteins, and to the DNA that carries the genetic blueprint for human development.

Free radicals have been linked to a whole gallery of woes: heart disease, Alzheimer's disease, atherosclerosis, mutations that can lead to cancer, problems with the body's immune system, and the process of aging itself. Conditions that increase free radicals are called pro-oxidant and those that counteract them are antioxidant.

The body has evolved to limit the damage free radicals can do. Every living cell in the body contains proteins known as enzymes, which speed up chemical reactions, and some of these enzymes are powerful antioxidants. There are also repair-and-clean-up enzymes that remove oxidized fatty-acid molecules from damaged membranes and damaged protein. There is a constant, dynamic balance within the body between free-radical formation and its breakdown by antioxidants.

Unfortunately, as we get older, this balance begins to lean more towards the pro-oxidant side. Excessive pro-oxidation is called "oxidative" stress, and it can have many causes. Among them are poor diet, heavy drinking, smoking, stress, pollution from traffic fumes and from industrial processes, overexposure to the sun, radiation treatment, and deficiencies or excesses in trace elements or vitamins. Even excessive exercise can lead to a build-up of free radicals, and many marathon athletes run without taking adequate antioxidants. Astronauts run a special risk of oxidative stress because of the forms of radiation encountered in space and because they are not shielded by Earth's atmosphere. Heavy ion particles can cause cancer, eye cataracts, and damage brain cells, so their diet is very rich in antioxidants.

The Body's Defenses

Glutathione, a powerful antioxidant produced naturally by the body, is used up in the process of reducing oxidation and needs to be replenished. It is diminished by inflammation, by infections, and by altitude, and its level drops after exercise, exposure to strong daylight sun, and radiation treatment.

It cannot be taken by mouth, because it is broken down by acid in the stomach. However, cysteine, glycine, and glutamine, the three amino acids from which glutathione is made, can be found in all health stores. Whey, the watery liquid left when milk forms curd, as in cheese-making, is a very rich source of amino acids. Drinking it is another way of increasing glutathione production.

Apha-lipoic acid is another of the body's natural antioxidant defenses. It is soluble in both fat and water and works by blocking the attachment of glucose to collagen, helping to keep blood vessels, skin, and joints from becoming stiff and inflexible.

Many more antioxidants can be found mostly in richly-colored fruits and vegetables. Look for foods that are bright orange, red, dark green, or blue. The best way to redress the oxidation balance is to manage what you eat and to include generous quantities of foods rich in antioxidants.

Vitamins and Trace Elements

A number of degenerative diseases associated with aging—among them heart disease, Alzheimer's, osteoarthritis, and cancer-have been shown to benefit from the antioxidants contained in vitamins and trace elements. Vitamins A, D, E, and K are fat-soluble, while the B and C vitamins are water-soluble. Fat-soluble vitamins are used slowly. They accumulate in the liver and the body uses them as needed. In the case of the water-soluble vitamins, the body uses what it needs and gets rid of any excess in the urine. A, C, and E are the most powerful antioxidant vitamins.

The body cannot make vitamin A on its own, but it can take the beta-carotene found in carrots and apricots and turn it into vitamin A. The B vitamins and folates in green vegetables, fruit, and liver help to reduce the risk of heart disease. Combinations of vitamin supplements and other antioxidants are now making their way into the market, and, more importantly, they are being prescribed by mainstream doctors. An example of this is the combination in pill form of vitamins A, B2 (riboflavin), C, E, and lutein and lycopene, together with some trace metals (trade name ICaps). This combination is recommended to keep eyes healthy as we age. It improves night vision and eye-dryness, particularly in post-menopausal women, and is said to stave off cataracts and to help in macular degeneration, a disorder that causes blurred vision and reduced color perception.

Trace elements are minerals such as magnesium, zinc, selenium, copper, manganese, and iron, which are required in minute amounts for healthy growth and development and for the absorption of some vitamins. Vitamin E, for instance, cannot be absorbed without the presence of the trace element selenium.

The body does not make these essential minerals, so we get them from the foods we eat or the supplements we take and the water we drink. Ultimately, they all come from the soil. Health spas became popular in ancient times when it was discovered that drinking the water from natural springs had beneficial side effects. Plants are rich sources of these trace elements and can provide all we need. Nuts are a particularly excellent source.

Nature's Treasure House of Antioxidants

There are many other sources of antioxidants. Water plants such as algae and kelp can play a role in keeping us healthy. Seaweed is a standard part of the Asian diet and is increasingly finding its way into the Western diet. The Japanese have a reputation for longevity, and this may have a good deal to do with what they eat. This includes the seaweed *nori*, the black paper-like sheet that is used to wrap rice and fish, *hijiki*, a shredded black seaweed; and various kelps, such as *wakame.*

In the USA, the microscopic algae *spirulin* and the fresh-water wild blue-green algae AFA (Aphanizomenon-Flos-Aquae), found in Lake Upper Klamath, in Oregon, are very rich in antioxidants, vitamins, and trace elements. Forty years ago, when the Soviet space program first started planning a manned trip to Mars, they experimented with growing algae on the spacecraft to provide a fresh source of food for this long trip. They believed that algae in the diet would give protection against space radiation, even though its antioxidant properties were not known at that time. Although the trip to Mars was delayed for the usual budgetary reasons, the antioxidant value of algae has now come into its own.

Wild spinach-type greens, kale, dandelion, mustard greens, and especially purslane—a small, succulent leaf creeper herb used in salads—provide strong antioxidants. They form the basis of the diet on the Greek island of Crete, whose inhabitants also claim to live long, healthy lives.

Drinking two to four cups of green tea a day has many beneficial health effects. Differences in the color and flavor of tea depend not just on the leaf but also on the way it is processed. Green tea is steam-heated or oven dried very quickly. Unlike black tea, which is dried slowly on racks so that it ferments and the leaves turn brown, green tea is not fermented. This leaves it with higher levels of antioxidants.

Perhaps the most often discussed antioxidant of all has been the glass of wine. A glass of red wine a day is now recommended for its antioxidant properties to "ward off the tooth of time." Though white wine has recently also been found to have antioxidant properties, these are not as high as in red wine attributed to the tannins found in the grape skin.

The U.S. Department of Agriculture (USDA) has come up with a scale of relative antioxidant value of common foods. The Oxygen Radical Absorbance Capacity, or ORAC, scale was developed by measuring blood antioxidants levels after eating 100 g of a food. Many of us have heard about the antioxidant value of blueberries but who had ever thought prunes would be even better. Prunes score highest at 5,770 compared to 2,400 for blueberries, 1,260 for spinach, and 739 for red grapes. More information can be found at the USDA database.

What You Can Do about It

Most of us have room to improve our diets. This is particularly true for adolescents and seniors. A recent USDA survey of people aged sixty-five to eighty-four found that only 21% ate a "good" diet, and in 12% of the cases sampled the diet was "very poor." The remaining 67% ate too much processed food and fast food.

The diet of adolescents is equally unhealthy. Fast food concessions are now to be found on many school premises, providing sugary treats such as doughnuts, Danish pastries, cookies, sugary cereals, packaged juices or soft drinks, pizza and hamburgers, bologna, and peanut butter and jelly sandwiches. Protein makes but a small proportion of the standard teenage diet. Salads are rare and fish even rarer.

Many factors influence our state of nutrition. It is not only what we eat that matters but when we eat and how much activity we take. We are bombarded with information about the latest diets, about food pyramids, about the correct proportions of fat, protein, and carbohydrate in the diet. But who wants to weigh or count every mouthful? Maybe the best advice was that given by Julia Child, one of America's most beloved chefs, on the occasion of her ninetieth birthday: "Eat a little bit of everything, but don't eat too much; small helpings and no snacks."

Timing Your Meals

Your metabolic rate—the rate at which your body produces energy—peaks first thing in the morning and gradually declines through the day. That does not necessarily mean you should have your biggest meal for breakfast, but it does mean that having a rich meal at night places an exacting burden on your body.

Try to time your meals so that they come before exercise, even if the exercise is only gardening, walking, or housecleaning. Eating before exercise, as long as it is a light meal, will ensure not only that you will have adequate endurance but that your body will not burn muscle as fuel—the opposite of what you are aiming for. Leave time, though, for the digestive process to get underway. For instance, eat a high-fiber, low-GI snack, such as a tuna sandwich or half a cup of nuts, one to two hours before strenuous exercise. And timing is important after such exercise as well: for maximum benefit in building muscle, eat a high-protein snack, such as whey or almonds, within thirty to ninety minutes of stopping your exercise.

A Little Goes a Long Way

"A little bit of what you fancy does you good" was the theme of a song by Cockney music-hall artist Marie Lloyd. It is said that when Jacqueline Kennedy ate out, she kept her figure by only ordering appetizer and dessert. There is a psychological benefit to eating something small but exquisitely tasty. If you crave chocolate, do not compromise. Read the label and select a very small piece of a chocolate that is high in cocoa liquor or mass and low in sugar content. Sugar is added to most chocolate to fool your taste buds and cover up for the absence of more expensive ingredients. With such a product, you are not tasting chocolate but sweet fat.

The Case for Chocolate

Chocolate has been much maligned. How could it possibly taste so good and also be good for you? Well, that is exactly what recent research is showing. Dark chocolate of the highest cocoa liquor and lowest fat content is rich in a class of compounds called flavanoids. These are believed to improve the function of blood vessels and prevent the buildup of cholesterol.

Mary Engler at the University of California Medical Center, in San Francisco, completed a randomized clinical trial on eleven people fed one and a half ounces of dark chocolate a day for two weeks When measured with ultrasound, the diameter of an artery in their arm (which are similar to those that supply the heart) was considerably greater in those who ate the dark chocolate than in the control group—and that is definitely a good thing!

Feed Your Mind—and Go for Color

The connection between food and the mind is very strong. Food is one of life's most pleasurable experiences, so make sure you savor it. Do not eat for the sake of eating, but eat food that looks, smells, and tastes delicious. Make the setting appealing. Do not eat on the run, in front of the TV, standing in the kitchen, or by the refrigerator. The French, renowned for their lengthy lunches, make a ritual of it, serving small portions with plenty of waiting time in between the many courses.

Enjoy the ritual of meals shared with good company and good music. Keep your dishes simple but varied, using vegetables or fruit in season, and serve food attractively. Decorate your kitchen with culinary art, using the green, yellow, red, and orange of fresh fruit and ready-to-eat vegetables. Change the culinary color scheme with the season, using the greens and reds of apples, the yellows of squashes, the warm color of oranges. Limes, tangerines, peppers, and cucumbers all have their shades and tints to add. Squeeze some tangerine peel to squirt some of its wonderful aroma into the room and lift your spirits. Grow some herbs on your windowsill. They smell good and are a living reminder to add them to your cooking.

A Medicine Cabinet in the Pantry

It just so happens that fruit and vegetables that are richest in the things best for us are the ones that have the brightest colors and most intense flavors. Helpful antioxidants are mostly to be found in dark green leafy vegetables such as spinach, kale, broccoli, Brussels sprouts, watercress, and sweet peppers. Greens such as broccoli, cabbage, and kale protect us from colon cancer.

Orange-colored food such as sweet potatoes and cantaloupe provide beta-carotene that builds the antioxidant vitamin A and may reduce the chance of atherosclerosis. Yellow corn is good for cataracts and macular degeneration. Bright-colored fruit such as tomatoes, peaches, cantaloupe, kiwi, and all the berries, blueberries and cranberries in particular, are packed with antioxidants. Tomatoes contain lycopene, which may prevent heart and lung disease and, when cooked, help to prevent prostrate cancer. Blueberries help protect against memory loss and other age-related changes in the brain. Kiwi fruit is claimed to be good for short-term memory and for balance. Though rich in color, carrots, grapes, apricots, oranges, and watermelon are not included in this list, because they have a high sugar content and an extremely high glycemic index.

And if you wonder how much of all these you should eat, seven or eight servings of fruit and vegetables a day should do it. Fresh is better than frozen unless the food is flash frozen. Read the label to make sure sugar has not been added to the frozen fruit.

Even in fish, color is a good indicator of nutritional value. Fish are a rich source of the essential fatty acids that we need all of our lives, and even so more as we age. The best fish for this purpose are the dark-colored oily fish, such as salmon, herrings, sardines, tuna, and mackerel, which are rich in omega-3 and omega-6. Wild salmon is by far the richest source of these two fatty acids, and the darker in color, the better. Eating oily fish is probably also good for the brain, just as your mother said. Fish, of course, is also a wonderful source of protein. But caution should be exercised to stay away from farmed fish where antibiotics are used in the breeding process.

The Defensive Diet

Reducing damage to your health does not mean cutting out all fats. The fats that do the damage are saturated animal fats and man-made fats, such as cooking fats and margarine, which have been hydrogenated—turned from liquid to solid by being drenched with hydrogen. Animal fats from a slice of the best beef come with unhealthy amounts of saturated fats that can cause damage when they find their way into the blood vessels of the brain. A "well-marbled" piece of steak is the most tasty, but it also contains the most fat. Lean meat from grass-fed cattle is best for us.

The meat eaten by our ancestors was game, and both hunter and prey stayed lean. Can we live without beef? Sure we can, but there is no harm in the occasional small lean steak. In general, though, if you want meat, stick with organic or free-range chicken, turkey, and game. Veal, pork, and well-trimmed lamb are leaner than most beef.

Manage What You Eat, but Don't Forget to Use Gravity

Manage what you eat and when you eat it. Variety is the key. Some foods are high in antioxidants and lower in vitamins or amino acids. Others are rich in omega-3 and low in something else. Ensure your body makes best use of what you eat by continuing to use gravity so that what you eat is better absorbed and your body produces its own antioxidants. These are the basic rules that will prevent the damage generated by bad eating habits. Remaining active is one of the best ways of achieving this goal.

Food is intended to give us pleasure, provide energy, build muscle, and keep bones strong. Vitamins and minerals are needed to ensure the chemical processes work well. Fiber will maintain the smooth functioning of intestines and slow down the absorption of starches. Antioxidants and anti-inflammatory agents will prevent cell damage. Remember to do whatever it takes to smooth out insulin spikes, and remember that calories do matter. However, for all that, the healthiest diet in the world, one that satisfies the taste buds and prevents damage to the body, will only work if we capitalize on gravity.

10

Lifespan

Psalm 90 tells us: "The days of our years are three score years and ten; and if by reason of strength they be four score years, yet is their strength labor and sorrow; for it is soon cut off, and we fly away." This is not too different from today's average lifespan for the populations of the developed world, which ranges from seventy to eighty years. Yet the Bible also looks back to a golden age, when life was measured, apparently, not in decades but in centuries.

According to the Book of Genesis, "All the days that Adam lived were nine hundred and thirty years," and he was still begetting children when he was more than 800 years old. The record seems to have been held by Adam's great, great, great, great, great grandson, Methuselah: "And all the days of Methuselah were nine hundred sixty and nine years." His name has become synonymous with longevity.

Incredible as these numbers may seem, we find ourselves once more in an era of genetic discoveries. Some scientists believe that, in theory at least, there is no compelling reason why human beings should not be able to live so long that centenarians will one day be regarded as striplings. This may sound far fetched, but it is a fact that the average lifespan has been steadily increasing. When it comes to longevity, humankind has good genes. John Wilmoth at the University of California, Berkeley, is quoted in Fred Warshofsky's *Stealing Time* as saying, "I don't think we can live forever, but we haven't yet been able to find a fixed limit for the human lifespan."

A longer lifespan assumes, of course, that we do not succumb to disease or allow time and neglect to bring on the symptoms that have become associated with aging. Neglect means adopting a lifestyle that ignores the fact that we live in a field of gravity, the force that pulls us down. The only way to remain healthy in this field is to stay within "normal limits," by refusing to be pulled down, by defying gravity rather than giving in to it. A vintage car may not be as nippy as it once was, but it can certainly win prizes in a *concours d'elegance*, appreciate in value, and in due course become a collector's item. It is the same with human beings: proper care can prolong active life. And it is an active, healthy life that most of us want, not the mere accumulation of years.

In addition to the right kind of care, people who set their sights on longevity need to start with the right heritage. We all know someone who has reached a "good age." Chances are, they have parents or relatives who lived for a long time as well. We expect their offspring will live long too. Is this a sign that they have learned good health habits, or was longevity passed along in their genes? Some, though not many, reach a good age despite their bad habits. Lifelong smokers and drinkers who have led very active lives and who have a sense of fun occasionally beat the odds. From decades of research, we know that astronauts who spend a long time away from the force of gravity show the same symptoms of disability when they return to Earth as those that afflict the elderly. But no such link has been established between gravity and the expectation of life. The consensus among scientists is that longevity lies in the genes. Thus, the search has begun for the gene, or genes, that confer long life.

The Oldest on Record

Although humans live longer than almost any other mammal, several animals and plants can outlive us. The oldest known living organism is one shrub, the King's Holly (*Lomatia tasmanica,*) found in the western region of Tasmania and recently carbon-dated as being around 43,000 years old. In terms of venerability, it easily beats the previous record-holder, the bristlecone pine (*Pinus longaeva*) of California, one specimen of which is known to have lived for 4,900 years.

In the world of water, the carp (*Cyprinus carpio*) has a reputation for longevity, but its lifespan of forty to fifty years is unimpressive compared with that of the bowhead whale *(Baleana mysticetus)*, which can live for 200 years or more. The bowhead also has the distinction of possessing the world's largest mouth—a chasm 16 ft long by 8 ft wide (5 m by 2.5 m). The Galapagos giant turtle (*Geochelone elephantopus*) can live for well over 100 years, and some individuals are believed to be more than 200 years old.

Elephants live roughly as long as humans. The oldest recorded was an Indian elephant *(Elephas maximus)* named Lakshimikutty, who died in 1997 at the age of eighty-four. Among humans, women tend to live several years longer than men, and longevity varies from nation to nation. Japan heads the league table with an expectation of life of 77.16 years for men and 84.01 for women (UN figures, calculated in 1999). It is not always possible to verify claims of longevity, because records may be unreliable, but the longest human life on authenticated record was that of the Frenchwoman Jeanne Louise Calment, who was born on February 21, 1875, and died on August 4, 1997, at 122 years, 164 days old.

The Choice: Reproduction or a Long Life?

How long we might live is genetically determined, since your genes predispose you to the diseases you may get along the way. One long-held theory was based on the belief that a person's lifespan was determined by his or her biological clock. There were just so many programmed cycles in a lifetime. But no clock-type genes have been discovered to support this theory. Another theory along similar lines is based on the turnover time of each cell in the body. If every seven years or so, every cell in the body is replaced by a copy of itself, there is always the possibility of something going wrong. What you get by the time you are aged seventy is a ninth copy taken from a series of copies, each of which may be inferior in some way to the one it replaced. Imagine the end result of such a process in a copying machine!

In trying to find out to what extent longevity is due to genes versus other factors, scientists have turned to simple organisms with short life spans. This allows many generations to be studied in a relatively short time. The first identification of a single gene that affects lifespan came in the early 1980s from work with a miniscule worm bearing the lovely name of *Caenorhabditis elegans*, which normally has a lifespan of fifteen to twenty days. This gene was appropriately named Age-1. One of the findings was that the worms that lost mobility earlier died younger. Other organisms used in this type of research are yeast, fruit flies (*drosophila*, which live about twenty-eight days), and mice (which live up to three years).

A relationship between longer life and late reproduction was first discovered in the study of fruit flies. In the 1950s, John Maynard Smith, a British engineer who designed fighter planes in World War II and later turned his attention to evolutionary biology, noticed that when females were rendered less fertile, they lived longer. Michael Rose at the University of California, in Irvine, followed up Smith's work in the 1980s. He found he could extend the life of fruit flies by delaying the age at which they first gave birth. In this way, fruit flies lived as long as ten weeks. Those who were still able to reproduce at later ages produced off-spring with much longer life spans. In effect, Rose selectively bred these new generations of fruit flies for longevity.

The genetic tradeoff between long life and lower fertility has also been explored in humans. In 1998, Thomas B. Kirkwood, while at the University of Manchester, and Rudi G. J. Westendorp, of Leiden University Medical Center, in the Netherlands, reported on the analysis of records of 13,667 married female British aristocrats born between 740 and 1875. They were chosen because better records were available for aristocrats. Those who had fewer children or gave birth to their first child later in life lived longer. Women who died between fifty and eighty gave birth to their first child at 24.3 and had an average of 2.4 to 2.6 children. Those who lived to between eighty and ninety had their first child past twenty-five and averaged 2.1 children. The women who lived into their nineties did not have their first child until about twenty-seven and had on average only 1.8 children.

Kirkwood went on to propose a theory of aging. If aging is a tradeoff between reproduction and long life, the body cells of those who put a lot of energy into giving birth and raising children would be left with less energy to devote to repair, maintenance, and stress menegement. Unrepaired imperfections that accumulate in cells over time result in the physical and mental erosion we associate with aging.

Cynthia Kenyon at the University of California, in San Francisco, dramatically extended the fifteen-to-twenty-day life of the worm *C. elegans* by removing its germ cells, which are needed for reproduction. This meant that the worm, much like eunuchs, who normally live longer than other males, did not have to devote metabolic energy to reproduction.

The Age-1 gene appears to shorten life, since the lifespan of *C. elegans* increased when the gene was eliminated. The lifespan of the worms can be extended by this means to thirty-three days on average, with some living to the ripe old age of forty-two days. What is more, they are resistant to the forms of stress that result from high temperatures or from the build-up of oxidation in the cells. Some forty other genes have been found to increase lifespan by at least 20%

in this worm. All life-extending genes also seem to confer stress-resistance, supporting the notion that stress resistance and longer life are strongly coupled.

Is There a Gene That Will Allow Us to Live Longer?

The race for a single longevity gene is a hot one. Which one of the forty genes identified will it be? Several biotechnology companies have supported university research programs or set up independently in the hope of some day creating drugs that will extend human life. DeCode Genetics, an Icelandic biotechnology company, claims to have identified the location of such a gene in humans. They did so by taking advantage of Iceland's unique birth and death records, which date all the way back to the time of the Vikings. They identified 1,200 long-lived individuals, some of them more than ninety years old, and found they were much more closely interrelated than another group who had lived only for the average number of years for the time. They excluded the possibility that it was their lifestyles that had made the difference, because Icelanders, a tightly-knit population of only 270,000 in the period under survey all had similar lifestyles. Kari Stefansson, chief executive officer of the company, believes long life is conferred by a single gene. She is quick to add she does not believe it can make you immortal, since we inherit other genes that predispose us to illnesses that can cut life short.

What seems clear is that there are many factors that determine how long we may live. They include genetic heritage and environmental or lifestyle factors. Stress, poor nutrition, injury, a disease can all shorten life.

Growing New Body Parts

The body has an innate capacity to repair and restore itself, and Mother Nature is now being helped by modern medical technology. It is possible, through the use of stem cells, to grow replacement tissues, such as bone marrow. Stem cells are the embryonic cells with which all babies start life in the womb. They are undifferentiated at the start, but each stem cell has the potential to develop according to the role it is called on to perform. One cell will become an eye cell, another a brain cell, yet another a message-carrying nerve cell, and so on. Because of the new technology that has arisen out of experiments in cloning, combined with stem-cell research, the day may not be too far away when it will be possible to replace many tissues that are aged or diseased. Some couples with an eye to the future are already having stem cells from the umbilical cords of their babies stored in special banks in preparation for the day when a life-giving transplant might be needed.

William Haseltine, chairman and chief executive officer of Human Genome Science Inc., in Rockville, Maryland, proposed the concept of "regenerative medicine." He asserts, "If the body wears out or is injured by trauma or disease, it can rebuild, replace, or restore the affected body part to its normal healthy function." In addition to using stem cells, organs made from a person's own tissue can now be grown outside the body for re-implantation. This has been done in laboratory animals and, in a few cases, in humans, to grow skin, bone, and ligaments. Replacement bladders, blood vessels, and heart valves are on the way. Even more interesting is the potential for using human genes, proteins, and antibodies to stimulate the body to correct a defect, instead of using drugs or organ replacement. Somebody who loses an arm or a leg might one day be able to grow a new one, if only we could understand how a newt can re-grow its severed tail. If we are to defeat the consequences of aging, we must do this kind of research to understand the processes of cell division, repair, replacement, injury, and death

The Life and Death of Cells

Throughout life, the cells of the human body, like those of any other living organism, die and are replaced by new ones. There are several ways in which the life of a cell can come to an end. The body may lose its ability to repair cells. A cell may, like its host organism, cease to reproduce, grow old, and die. Or it may at any age be sacrificed for the good of the organism, via a suicidal process called "programmed cell death" or *apoptosis* (from the Greek "to fall off"). Cells can also perish if they are displaced or starved by immortal cells—cancer cells. These killer cells do not die themselves until they have destroyed their host. Understanding why and how cancer cells can live for ever, given adequate nourishment, is a fascinating topic of research for scientists who study aging.

Unlike cancer cells, which can divide indefinitely, normal cells in the body eventually stop dividing—a stage called *senescence*. In other words, when a cell stops dividing it becomes *old*. Researchers have found that cells grown outside the body in a culture that supplies them with nutrients can live in non-dividing senescence for years before dying, as long as they are provided with fresh culture medium every week. The number of times a young cell divides in culture is directly related to the longest lifespan of the organism from which it came. Cells from mice, which live up to three years, divide ten times or less before becoming senescent, whereas those from the centenarian Galapagos giant turtle divide as many as 130 times before senescence. Cells from patients with the premature aging disease known as Werner's syndrome go through many fewer divisions when grown in culture than those from a normal person of the same age.

The problem with senescent cells is that not only do they no longer divide, but they become a liability. They can malfunction, and unlike normal cells that malfunction, they will not commit suicide. As senescent cells accumulate, they begin to put out chemicals that cause inflammation and the breakdown of surrounding tissue. Skin, for instance, becomes wrinkled, and cuts and bruises do not heal as well or as fast. Eventually, when the cell dies, it swells up and bursts, spilling its contents. Released enzymes then trigger more inflammation, which kills neighboring cells. A vicious cycle of inflammation and tissue damage is underway.

What causes cells to stop dividing seems to be the shortening of a portion of DNA (the carrier of genetic information) that protects the tips of chromosomes (the thread-like structures in the cell nucleus). Chromosomes carry the genes that determine sex and pass on the characteristics a baby inherits from its parents. Researchers called these chromosome tips *telomeres*, which is Greek for "end portion." They observed that each time a cell divided, a small portion at the end of the telomeres broke off. Eventually, the telomeres shortened so much that there was nothing left to divide. In essence, telomeres were clocking cell time.

However, some cells in humans, such as sperm cells, egg cells, and cancer cells, do not become senescent. They continue to divide, because their telomere tips keep being replaced. The same thing happens to all cells in the bodies of non-mammalian species. Researchers discovered that an enzyme, which they called *telomerase*, was responsible for replacing telomere tips. In humans and other mammals, the gene that produces telomerase is switched off after a certain number of cell divisions. Would switching on this telomerase gene increase the risk of cancer? Jerry Shay and Woodring Wright at the University of Texas Southwestern Medical Center, in Dallas, discovered a way to switch on the telomerase gene in human cells. This resulted in 280 divisions instead of the 50-division limit originally recorded for normal human cells. The commercial potential of this discovery spawned the formation of the biotechnology company Geron Corporation, in Menlo Park, California. Collaboration between Geron scientists and Wright and Shay had human cells dividing and doubling well over 400 times.

The good news is that this phenomenal extension of a cell's dividing life did not result in cells that looked or grew like cancer cells. But the ability to restore telomeres to their youthful length does not yet imply we can rejuvenate the entire body. The possibility that a telomerase-treated cell might become malignant at some stage downstream must first be ruled out. It could take a while before telomerase finds applications in postponing humankind's sunset years.

In the meantime, there is a good chance that it could be used to rejuvenate specific cells, for example, in the body's immune system. Imagine if, like taking an annual flu shot, people over sixty could get a telomerase gene boost to their immune systems. Many older people who would otherwise die from pneumonia and other infections might reach today's 120-year limit. Ways of introducing telomerase into skin cells are already being developed. Barring unforeseen complications, telomerase creams and lotions will undoubtedly join the ranks of rejuvenating cosmetics in the next few years. Not only could life be longer, it could also be wrinkle free!

Programmed cell death, or *apoptosis*, is very different from the death of a senescent cell. This happens even as the embryo is forming. Apoptosis provides a way to remove unwanted cells during growth and development and to defend against viral infection. It is also one way in which the body protects itself against cancer and genetic damage. Normal cells have a genetic suicide program that tells them when it is time to die. If they are damaged or abnormal or in the wrong place at the wrong time, their apoptosis program eliminates them by literally digesting the cell from the inside out. For instance, during the development of the nervous system, numerous nerve cells are formed. In order to connect with other nerve cells, muscles, eyes, or ears, they send out shoots that track chemical signals from the cells they are trying to reach. If, for some reason, the nerve shoot goes astray, the cell initiates its suicide program.

Cell death by apoptosis, unlike slow death by senescence, does not damage surrounding cells and tissue or cause inflammation. Once a cell has initiated its cell-death program, it changes shape, shrivels, begins to break up, and is finally engulfed and digested or cleared through the blood, to be eliminated from the body through normal excretion. There are many genes and stimuli that can initiate the apoptosis program as well as others that prevent it from happening. The immune system works by sending its killer cells to induce infected cells to commit suicide. Some viruses carry genes that block the suicide of the host cells. In this way, the virus is able to thrive, multiply, and spread within the body.

Apoptosis can also trigger the formation of healthy new cells. New cell formation in the brain has been shown to follow on the heels of apoptosis. Jeffrey Macklis, at Harvard's Children's Hospital, showed that triggering apoptosis in a specific part of the brain cortex stimulates stem cells to become mature adult brain cells. The required new cells are formed only in the damaged area.

Could Eating Less Prolong Life?

The oldest theory regarding lifespan revolves around the notion of *how fast we live*. The concept is based on the premise that we have a fixed total metabolic credit that is used up over a lifetime. The faster the metabolic rate, the shorter the life span. This theory was put to the test by Clive McCay at Cornell University, in New York, in 1935. Simply by cutting back the amount of calories in the diet to near-starvation levels—*caloric restriction*—he found he could extend the lives of rats by 50%. These results were ignored for decades, until the early 1970s, when Roy Walford at UCLA began repeating them in mice. After hundreds of experiments, mice that were fed 40% fewer calories, but with all the nutrients they needed, consistently lived one-third longer than their counterparts who ate all they wanted.

Though Walford's research was first deemed something of an oddity, it has since been recognized as central to understanding the mechanisms of longevity. It is now established that reducing the consumption of calories always leads to a longer life, whether the organism is a single cell, fly, worm, mouse, or rat. Rick Weindruch at the University of Wisconsin Regional Primate Center is studying our genetic cousins, rhesus monkeys, which live to about thirty to thirty-five years of age, and is about halfway through the experiment. The monkeys on caloric restriction are already showing the same healthy symptoms as those revealed in other experiments. Time alone will tell whether they will also live longer.

Lean Times in the Biosphere

I first met Roy Walford, the man who dramatically extended the life of mice by cutting down on their caloric intake, in 1988, when I went with a group from NASA's Ames Research Center, in California, to visit the Biosphere project in the desert outside Tucson, Arizona. Biosphere, a domed structure covering three acres, was meant to be self-sufficient and provide an Earth-like ecosystem, including ocean, marshland, farmland, tropical forest, and desert, as well as edible plants and animals. Eight people lived in the sphere. Walford was medical officer for the project, responsible for the health and welfare of the other three men and four women participants. We at NASA were interested in what we could learn from Biosphere about building self-sufficient life-support systems and habitats. We also wanted to know what could be expected of human behavior during a long trip and stay on Mars. The Biosphere was much larger than anything we visualized for Mars, but I believed the information would be relevant.

In 1991, the doors were closed on Biosphere and its eight-member crew, who ranged in age from twenty-eight to sixty-seven (Walford's age at the time). The experiment lasted six months. Despite many years of careful planning, food production fell short of the requirements of the crew. Walford, with his research background and personal interest in caloric restriction, saw this as an opportunity. Like it or not, the Biosphere crew lived on a diet of only 1,800 calories a day. This is about 40% less than the 2,500 to 3,500 calories the average American eats daily. However, Walford made sure that what they ate was of high nutritional value. Together with the hard physical work of keeping Biosphere running, the participants were initially hungry but became increasingly lean and fit. Even more remarkable, they were getting healthier—much like the mice had in Walford's lab studies. They had less body fat, while their cholesterol, blood sugar, and blood pressure decreased. The number of white blood cells fell, indicating a stronger immune system. The crew showed the same physiological reactions to restricting calories as had the mice. Walford himself has been on a 1,700-calorie-a-day nutrient-rich diet for the last fourteen years. This is 30% less than the average intake for a man his size and age. He expects to add fifteen to twenty years to his life.

The calorie-restricted diet is gaining followers among those looking for the fountain of youth. However, as with any other diets, going overboard is always a danger. This is especially true when the diet is self-monitored and the vital importance of adequate nutrition is overlooked. At present, there is insufficient data to determine just how many fewer calories are needed to extend a healthy human life, not to mention what the drawbacks might be. Laura Johannes, writing in the *Wall Street Journal* in 2002, told of an on-line chat group of about 800 followers worldwide who call themselves "Cronics" and whose philosophy is: "Calorie Restriction with Optimal Nutrition." One member reports eating only 1,500 calories a day. Another, a thirty-seven-year-old man, is 5 ft 8 in tall and weighs 127 lb. His photograph shows a distinctly skeletal figure. Not surprisingly, perhaps, reports are apparently already coming in of reduced testosterone levels and abated interest in sex, lower body temperatures, and early signs of osteoporosis and anemia. Given our present state of knowledge, a restricted diet is not necessarily better for everyone.

There is a classic tale of Nasruddin Haj, the Turkish folklore character who scraped a living by picking firewood in the woods then loading it on his donkey and taking it to market to sell. Trying to figure out how to increase his net profit, he hit upon the novel idea of slightly reducing the amount of food he gave his donkey to eat. He was pleasantly surprised when the donkey seemed to work just as well as before. So he rationed the food still further, yet the animal continued to perform well. Delighted with his newly found source of wealth, he cut back still further on the food. To his chagrin, the donkey then died. The moral to this tale: too much economy, in the diet as in other matters, may not be such a good thing.

Scientists have been perplexed by the question of exactly how caloric restriction delays the changes associated with aging and extends both average and maximum lifespan in animals. The rhesus monkeys studied in Weindruch's research, for instance, had lower metabolic rates, lower blood sugar, and lower insulin levels as a result of their calorie-restricted diets. The glucose metabolism of the monkeys was vastly improved: their insulin was more efficient in getting glucose into cells where it is used and in removing it from the bloodstream. The same pleasing results are seen in very active persons who are not on calorie restriction, such as the members of a super-fit Norwegian ski-patrol team tested in the 1960s. So, it appears that calorie restriction works in the same way as increased activity in improving the sensitivity of cells to insulin. Rhesus monkeys can and do get diabetes with age, but none on caloric restriction have so far developed the disease.

If glucose is not effectively cleared from the bloodstream it sticks to hemoglobin in the red blood cells, reducing its ability to carry oxygen. Glucose also binds to the proteins, elastin, and collagen, in joints, skin, and muscle, causing them to stiffen. Toughening and stiffening of joints and skin are familiar consequences of aging. This process is accelerated by even a slight increase in body temperature. The lowering of body temperature by means of caloric restriction may be one factor in extending lifespan. It is recognized that a lower body temperature results in reduced oxygen consumption, a reduction in hormones produced by the thyroid, and a slowing down of the metabolism. Raj Sohal at Southern Methodist University, in Dallas, Texas, noticed that houseflies lived twice as long when the temperature was cooled down to 18° C. In a warm room (30° C), the flies increased their metabolism, used up more oxygen, and shortened their lives.

Researchers are converging on the unifying theme that caloric restriction works by reducing a high metabolic rate and so reducing damage from oxidation. Oxygen is essential to staying alive, but, paradoxically, it can also be hazardous to health. When the body burns oxygen to create energy, the unstable molecules known as free radicals are among the by-products. They can cause extensive damage to cell membranes, to DNA, and to many proteins. The greater the number of free radicals, the shorter the life of the organism. Conversely, anything that produces antioxidants retards this damage and extends life. Mice and rats on calorie-restricted diets have fewer free radicals and suffer less oxidative damage to cell membranes.

With humans on an all-you-can-eat diet, the highest oxidative damage occurs to cells in the brain, heart, and muscles—areas that are usually the prime targets of arthritis and other age-related degenerative diseases. The greatest benefit of caloric restriction is most obvious in these same tissues and is evident within a few weeks. This means that there are benefits in watching what you eat, even if you do not start until later in life. The most important thing is to make sure your diet is always rich in the necessary nutrients and antioxidants. Fortunately, science is coming to the rescue. Caloric restriction may not be the only answer to a longer life. Synthetic antioxidant drugs have recently been shown to extend the life of the worm *C. elegans* by 50%, while similar studies in mice are also showing promise.

What Part Does Gravity Play?

Gravity—or rather its absence or reduction—plays a key role in the development of aging symptoms, but whether it has any effect on lifespan is unknown at present. Gravity imposes a load on the body that can be reduced by going into space (or by taking to one's bed) and increased by centrifugation (spinning rapidly on a special apparatus). Because hypergravity increases the weight of the body, it is reasonable to expect that metabolism would be increased and longevity might be decreased. Indeed, fruit flies that lived their entire lives at higher gravity showed a tendency to die earlier. They also displayed reduced activity earlier in life—a symptom of aging. Rats that lived in 2 G conditions also had higher metabolic rates, higher oxygen consumption, and a greater glucose uptake. They were smaller but had less fat tissue, and their muscles and bones were stronger. Their lives were 6 to 10% shorter.

By contrast, living weightless for many months in space results in lower metabolism, lower body temperature, lower production of thyroid hormones, weaker muscles and bones, and a shift from muscle to fat.

While they are getting used to living and working in space, astronauts initially use up more energy. As they stay longer in space, they actually use 40% less energy than they would doing equivalent activities on Earth—simply because they do not have to work against gravity.

The Martian Lifespan?

There are no reliable data on longevity in space. Experiments carried out on the International Space Station and on the Russian space station *Mir* have not yet addressed this question, since they have not had the facilities to do multiple-generation studies. The aging-like symptoms associated with spaceflight have led many to assume aging is accelerated in space and lifespan is likely to be shortened. But the average lifespan of an astronaut, barring accidents, is certainly no lower than that of the rest of us. The aging symptoms are appropriate adaptations to reduced gravity. They only become a problem after the return from space. And once one is back in Earth's gravity, they are reversible.

Were human beings to live permanently in the lower gravity of Mars, the lifespan of those who survive and adapt completely to the new gravity conditions—0.6G—would be extended beyond Earth's limits, though it might take a few generations to see this happen.

11

So, What Is Aging?

There is no precise definition these days of aging or of old age. As jazz musician George William Curtis put it, "Age is a matter of feeling, not of years." You may have a picture in your mind of what an "old" person is—a wrinkled face, gray hair, poor eyesight and worse hearing, stooped posture, false teeth, failing memory—but you cannot reliably guess how old this person may be. Fifty years ago, some of these symptoms might have been seen in a forty or fifty-year-old, whereas today even a person who has turned eighty may not show most of them.

Shakespeare, who died in 1616, aged fifty-three, described the seven ages of man as ending in the pitiable state of second childhood: "Sans teeth, sans eyes, sans taste, sans everything." Today, you could describe some people over the age of one hundred as being "old" without necessarily implying that they have outlived their usefulness. Many centenarians have given abundant evidence of their liveliness. The number of candles on the birthday cake tells us nothing about how old a person looks or feels.

When the American Association of Retired Persons was formed in 1958, they defined a "senior" as somebody who had turned fifty. And a recent report by the Centers for Disease Control, in Atlanta, Georgia, referred to seniors and elderly people as those "fifty and older." These definitions are anachronistic, and so is the attitude of those who wrote them. Yet the attitude persists. If you are a forty-year-old writer in Hollywood, you are "over the hill." Actresses over forty have a hard time getting a good part. Being passed over for promotion or downsized at fifty in some organizational reshuffle is a fairly common experience.

The Mother Who Walked Out

Perceptions of what an "older" person is, and of what that person can and cannot do, have become so ingrained that people do not always realize that they are being condescending. A daughter takes her mother to the doctor for some minor ache. The doctor addresses his explanations to the daughter rather than to the mother directly, as if she is incapable of understanding, like a child. One Mother's Day, I saw a waiter do something like this at a restaurant, after which the elegant mother got up and walked out, much to the dismay of the family.

Clothes designed for the older woman can best be described as drab. Only recently have the Sporting Goods Manufacturers Association, in North Palm Beach, Florida, taken the lead in testing brighter, more appealing lines. Do TV companies not realize that advertisements for dentures and incontinence diapers will often cause their "senior" viewers to switch to another channel? Attitudes tend to be patronizing and condescending, with market researchers, who may well be recent graduates with little experience of life beyond the campus, deciding what older people want to see and what is best for them.

How Old Is Old?

Defining "old" becomes even more of a challenge as average lifespan steadily increases and as disabilities among at least some of the older groups decrease. Peter Peterson, deputy chairman of the Federal Reserve Bank of New York, described in 1999 those aged sixty-five to eighty-four as "young old" and those over eighty-five as "old old."

Thomas Perls, director of the New England Centenarian Study at Beth Israel Deaconess Medical Center, in Boston, defines the "oldest old" as being over ninety-five. Describing some of the centenarians he has met, he wrote, "In their nineties, they were essentially problem free. As nonagenarians, many were employed, were sexually active, and enjoyed the outdoors and the arts."

Sex and Aging

Active seventy and eighty-year-olds were once thought too frail to have sex, but surveys now show that healthy and enjoyable sex can still form part of their lives. Actors Tony Randall and Anthony Quinn were living testaments to the fallacy of setting age limits to reproductive capacity. Randall, who died in 2004 at age eighty-four and had a daughter at sev-

So, What Is Aging? 241

enty-three and a son at seventy-four, maintained when he was seventy-nine: "It's never too late to be a father." Quinn, who died at age eighty-six in 2001, fathered his twelfth child at seventy nine and a son at eighty-one.

Claims that an active sex life helps to keep you young date back to the Ancient Greeks, but they are based on anecdotal evidence rather than scientific proof. Spanish scientist Jaime Miquel, working with fruit flies at NASA's Ames Research Center, California, in the sixties, showed convincingly that male flies which had daily sex with a virgin female maintained their youthful vigor well beyond their siblings who were not sexually active. A hard act to follow, and not an easy experiment to confirm in humans!

Nevertheless, the results of a survey of the sex lives of 918 men aged forty-five to fifty-nine, followed up ten years later and published December 1997 in the *British Medical Journal*, tend to support the premise that sexual activity promotes a longer life. The death rate for the least sexually active men—those having fewer than one orgasm per month—was twice as high as that for the most active—those having two or more orgasms a week. New drugs such as Viagra are already extending the age limits for this important aspect of being human.

I think of those over eighty as falling into two general groups—those who are active participants in society and those who are not. The *active old* may be eighty, ninety, or a hundred but do not exhibit the appearance, behavior, or physical changes associated with their chronological age. They are usually physically active and have probably been so all their lives. Above all, they have developed excellent coping skills.

Holding the Years at Bay

The Outer Packaging

Most of us focus on how we look as the measure of aging. Hair dyes, laser treatment for wrinkles, exfoliating acid scrubs, electrical stimulation, spas, facials, expensive hormone-containing face creams, hair transplants, and plastic surgery promise much to both sexes. They have done wonders at keeping the outer packaging looking as young as possible.

Nips and tucks and skin-stretching to reverse the effects of gravity and time on drooping bums, breasts, cheeks, eyelids, and double chins are no longer just for

Hollywood stars and celebrities. Ordinary men and women as young as thirty are now candidates. Nor is it unusual to submit to the knife more than once in a lifetime. The result is often an expressionless face that looks like an astronaut's stretched "moonface" in space, caused by the fluid shifting upward in the absence of gravity.

Though wrinkles and other signs of aging, especially in men, have been accepted as signs of maturity and experience, vanity and the heavy emphasis on youth in our culture have driven many beyond plastic surgery. Botox injections can now be used to paralyze nerves and smooth away furrowed brows. Silicone implants give the appearance of voluptuous breasts. Collagen injections puff up lips.

Liposuction sucks away bulges of fat wherever they may have settled. Whatever the risk, the pain, and the price, presenting a more youthful exterior must seem worthwhile to those who have it done.

However, whether you are thirty or eighty, no plastic surgeon or make-up artist can give you that twinkle in the eye and the zest for life that project youthfulness. This depends on you.

The Inner Works

There is a more natural way of holding back the years. Let us start with the face, the part of our body that most directly expresses personality and that most people notice first. Unused facial muscles give in to gravity just like any other muscle in the body. Here is where gravity, used to strengthen face and neck muscles, can come to the rescue once again. Have you noticed how opera divas and actresses, who must articulate their lines clearly, do not show the sagging cheeks of non-singers of similar age? Singing, whistling, reading out loud, and elocution exercises are wonderful and enjoyable fitness training for facial muscles.

Maintaining or rebuilding the internal engine is more complex than looking after the outer appearance. Some people, by choice or through necessity, seek help from science. Injections of cells from sheep embryos have long been offered by European clinics as *rejuvenation therapy*. Replacement parts can be animal, such as pig-heart valves or human kidneys. They can be grown in a test tube or they can be artificial. Dr Christiaan Barnard, a South African surgeon, pioneered human heart-transplant surgery in 1967. Transplants of kidneys, livers, corneas, and heart-lung transplants have since been made possible.

The development of new synthetic materials, in particular metal alloys and synthetic polymers, has led the way to artificial replacements for heart valves, knees, hips, and teeth. Researchers are now working on programs to develop artificial retinas for the eye and titanium ears for the inner parts that do the hearing. Only twenty years ago, people who had to undergo cataract surgery had to remain very still in bed for days after the operation. It is now an outpatient procedure, performed with lasers under a local anesthetic.

The Need for Proper Maintenance

A well-tuned engine does not come out of a bottle. No single pill will keep us young. Stress management, vitamins, plenty of water, proper nutrition, and a daily glass of red wine may all play their part in maintaining the body's systems, but the best way to keep going is simply to keep going.

At a press briefing just before he went back into space in 1998, at the age of seventy-seven, John Glenn reinforced this message: "You are never too young to start exercising, but it is never too late to start." He referred to his elderly neighbor who "doesn't want to rust out" but "wants to burn out." Most of us would agree with Glenn and his neighbor. It is better to live a full, dynamic life with dignity than to clock up a few more years at the cost of one's independence and vitality.

Much younger than Glenn, but senior by AARP's definition, "Story" Musgrave flew on the Shuttle for the third time in 1993. At the age of fifty-eight he ventured outside to perform the repair work that saved the Hubble telescope.

For the rest of us, gardening, house cleaning, making the bed, walking up and down the stairs instead of taking the elevator, and walking to the store instead of driving are all simple ways of staying active. But as good as these activities may be, they are not enough by themselves to keep the body young. What we all need is to develop a varied and comprehensive set of gravity-using habits that specifically tone up every part and system of our bodies.

Make Friends with Gravity

We live in gravity. Our weight is a function of gravity. Those who aspire to a firm body by exercising with weights owe their benefits to gravity as well. Gravity affects the way we look, feel, and function.

So why do some people think of gravity as the enemy, as something bad that makes their bodies droop and sag? The truth is that if we let it drag us down, it will. But we humans are designed by evolution to use gravity as a stimulus to keep us Earth-healthy. Take it away, as in space, or do not use it fully on Earth and the symptoms of aging manifest quickly. Lying down during the day is a way of giving in to gravity, drastically reducing its impact. A gradual surrender to gravity is what happens to most of us throughout the course of our lives.

Exercise Is Not the Whole Story

Exercise can help to prevent or delay some of these symptoms. But just as diet alone will not keep you healthy, it is equally fallacious to believe that exercise alone or only one type of exercise or activity is the ultimate answer.

In space, hours of daily exercise in the absence of gravity proved to be almost useless in terms of preserving muscle mass and bone density, and balance and coordination were still impaired on return to Earth. After more than forty years of spaceflight, the Russians, the Europeans, the Japanese, and the Americans have all failed to find a wholly effective way of preventing the negative age-like symptoms astronauts show when they are deprived of the loading provided by gravity. Somehow, it is the totality of gravity's effect on the body that holds the key.

So what is the difference between simple exercise and harnessing gravity? In most instances, gravity makes exercise more effective. That is why exercise with weights or exercise that uses the weight of the body is so profitable. It is also why obese people have stronger bones. Often, of course, it is not a question of either exercise or gravity. Many activities combine the two—standing up, for instance, is an exercise that relies completely on living in gravity for its benefits.

Taking the concept of combining exercise with gravity further, the lessons learned from research into animals living at twice Earth's gravity separates the role of gravity from that of activity. Mice living for eight weeks on a centrifuge at 2 G ate more and were much less active but were considerably leaner and fitter than their brothers and sisters living in 1 G. They lost as much as 55% of their body fat. Gravity rather than activity alters metabolism to produce a leaner state. But they are complementary.

Living at 2 G may not sound practical for the average person. But it is not necessary to live at this higher G level all the time. I believe that daily exposure to hypergravity, on a centrifuge for short periods of time, may be all that is needed. I have designed just such a centrifuge, primarily as a means of keeping astronauts healthy on their way to Mars and back. Though not yet available to the public, it is used to expose research volunteers to higher G loads here on Earth, in effect exercising them at higher G loads. I think of it as whole-body weight training. It should accelerate bone and muscle repair in cases where people cannot exercise, either because of injury from sports, age, or disability. It could be used to shift metabolism to that leaner state where a person can eat more and yet lose body fat, as laboratory mice did. Charles Knapp at the University of Kentucky has begun evaluating this approach in healthy volunteers. It holds enormous promise.

How We Dodge Gravity in Our Daily Lives...

We spend a lot of time sitting. As the years go by, we adopt a lifestyle that requires us to use gravity less. In fact, we forget to use it altogether. Many of our daily activities—driving a car, watching TV, working in an office, or spending time in front of a computer screen—conspire to reduce the amount of time we spend interacting with gravity. So we reduce its influence.

...and Learning to Harness It

Exercise is commendable, but it is only part of the solution. You need to know which exercises use gravity best, because different exercises produce different benefits. You need to become informed in order to make smart choices. Remember to stand up often. Activities that use weights—hand-held or the body's own—involve the all-important element of working against gravity.

The Threat That Looms over Our Children

Physical education is a low priority in public schools. It has all but disappeared from the curriculum of all states, except for Illinois. Unless organized or encouraged by parents and communities outside school hours, many children would participate in almost no structured exercise activity. When our children are not eating or sitting at their desks, they are not necessarily participating in some sport or outdoor activity. They are increasingly likely to be slouched in front of the TV or a computer. The President's Council on Physical Fitness in Washington, D.C., is deeply concerned about this trend. Poor eating habits and lack of exercise at this critical time of development hamper the proper growth of bone and muscle and have a damaging effect on metabolism, motor coordination, and brain function.

The effects are even more dramatic in children than in healthy adults who become inactive later in life. And they may not be reversible, since experiences during development frequently have permanent consequences. Sad though it may be, some trend-forecasters believe that today's young people may be the first generation in decades to have a lower life expectancy than their parents. Depending on what data you choose to consider, 20–50% of school-age children in the U.S. are already obese, making them prime targets for many diseases. Late-onset Type-2 diabetes, once not expected to appear until around the age of fifty or over, is now affecting some people in their teens, twenties, and thirties. The not-for-profit Rand Corporation in Santa Monica, California, concluded in 2002 that obesity shortens lifespans by twenty years.

Gravity Knows No Age

The message of this book is for the young just as much as it is for those of advancing years. It is not enough to find the formula that enables only the elderly to be active, healthy, and independent as long as they live. We must recognize that as long as we live in Earth's gravity, the same formula applies for all of us, at all ages. Aging begins the day we are born, and it can be accelerated or slowed down according to the way we live.

The famous researcher Madame Curie remarked, "Nothing in life is to be feared. It is only to be understood." The sooner we understand and appreciate how our body was designed and adapted to sense and respond to stimuli such as light, temperature, sound, taste, touch, and gravity, the better off we will be. Though we know much about all these senses, the importance of gravity as the crucial stimulus to healthy living, as we have learned from our experience in space, has not been fully understood.

The Mice That Cannot Swim

The positive influence of gravity affects every system in the body. It loads bones, muscles, and joints with weight, and so keeps them strong and healthy. It keeps systems tuned and responsive by stimulating the senses, controlling blood pressure, setting the body clock, and alerting the nervous system. So far, we know only very little about how gravity is sensed and communicated to these systems. The vestibular system of the inner ear, the system that regulates balance, seems to be a primary player. Once more, the study of mice revealed a surprising insight.

Chuck Fuller and his group at the University of California, at Davis, studied a genetic strain of mice born without vestibular hair cells. These animals appear generally normal except that their heads are slightly tilted, they do not respond to linear acceleration, and they cannot swim. Normal mice are excellent swimmers.

Since the vestibular system of the inner ear is known to be a primary receptor of gravity, they wanted to know how animals, in which the gravity receptor function was selectively eliminated, would respond to living at 2 G. The researchers were surprised to find that these mice showed none of the changes they had recorded before in normal mice living at 2 G. They did not eat less, were not less active, nor did they lose body fat. And their circadian rhythms and regulation of body temperature were just as if they had been living at 1 G all the time.

From this and subsequent work, the researchers proposed an intriguing theory. Gravity does not act on each system separately. As the primary gravity receptor, the vestibular system is central to the actions of gravity in *all* body systems and functions. When it works properly, it sends messages, through projections, to other parts of the brain in order to generate appropriate responses. When it does not, a number of clinical disorders result, including disturbances of the body clock and metabolism, fitful sleep-wake cycles, anxiety, and dysfunction of the autonomic system, which among other things regulates blood pressure.

Life Goes On...and On

It is an undeniable fact that people in the developed world are living longer. In 1991, the National Center for Health Statistics reported an amazing 50% increase in life expectancy in the U.S. during the twentieth century. And the curve is getting steeper. In the 1950s, the average life expectancy at birth was fifty-one. In 1991, it had grown to seventy-three for white men, sixty-five for black men, eighty for white women, and seventy-four for black women. The most recent U.S. census of 2000 tells us that the average life expectancy at birth is 73.9 years for men and 79.6 years for women. Research into the causes of aging has identified genes that increase longevity. Scientists now talk of lifespans of 150 by 2050.

The World's Oldest Human Beings

According to the 2005 *Guinness Book of Records*, 114-year-old Hendrijke Van Andel-Schipper, born in June 1890 in the Netherlands, is now the world's oldest person. On March 2004, Fred Hale Sr. from Syracuse, New York, who was born December 1, 1890, became the oldest man in the world at the age of 113 years and 95 days.

The record for the oldest man (121 years) was formerly held by Japanese Shigechiyo Izumi (1865–1986) and for the oldest woman (122 years) by Jeanne Calment in France (1875–1997). The *Guinness Book* researchers have on file just over forty supercentenarians—people over the age of 110 now living. Living beyond 113 is extremely rare.

People over eighty-five, having survived or escaped most diseases, are often healthier and more active than many who are younger. The number of Americans aged one hundred or more has doubled since 1980, and four out of five of them are women. There are at present 50,000 centenarians across the United States, and the projection forecasts that by 2050 there will be around 1 million. In France, there are 1.2 million people over eighty-five and 7,662 centenarians, compared with 200 in 1953.

Congratulations from the Queen...6,500 Times

It is not just in the United States and France that the number of centenarians has been increasing sharply in the past few decades. The same trend can be seen in every part of the developed world. Queen Elizabeth II makes the one hundredth birthday of her subjects an extra special day by sending them a congratulatory telegram with the royal crest at its head. It reads "I AM SO PLEASED TO KNOW THAT YOU ARE CELEBRATING YOUR HUNDREDTH BIRTHDAY ON [THE APPROPRIATE DATE IS INCLUDED HERE]. I SEND MY CONGRATULATIONS AND BEST WISHES TO YOU ON SUCH A SPECIAL OCCASION."

The telegram, carrying a full-color photograph of the smiling Queen, goes to those who join the ranks of centenarians in every Commonwealth country where she is acknowledged as the head of state—a group that includes countries with populations as large as those of the United Kingdom, Australia, Canada, and New Zealand and as small as those of the Solomon Islands and Tuvalu. In 1953, the first full year of her reign, the Queen sent out 274 such telegrams. In 2002, there were just under 6,500.

Investigators studying centenarians note that although these people suffered their share of life's blows, they have been successful in overcoming them. Apart from good genes and good stress management, centenarians were optimistic, cheerful, and determined, with a great will to live, thinking of others and staying in touch with family, friends, and loved ones. French gerontologist Francoise Forette believes that by adopting such attitudes, "anyone can put off the inevitable, even if we do not have a centenarian's genes."

Tom Perls at the Medical Center, in Boston, is amazed by the vitality of centenarians he has met. He describes them as usually lean in build, non-smoking, with a happy-go-lucky personality and the ability to manage their stress well. Most have family members enjoying a long life, which points to good genes. He sees them as a "pot of gold" of information, possessing amazing genetic secrets about aging that could lead to new treatments. To make sure you enjoy your later years, keep on defying gravity, do not neglect your exercise, do not neglect your diet, and above all, do not neglect your family and friends.

Lessons from Other Lands

We have much to learn from different cultures about how best to encourage healthy and active aging. The tradition of four generations living under one roof family, once common in China, Japan, and India, is gradually disappearing as the younger members move to the city or overseas, chasing new opportunities or escaping a hierarchy in which the mother-in-law ruled the roost.

In the Land of Shangri-La

Surrounded by the jagged, snow-capped peaks of the Karakorum Mountains of northern Kashmir, in a region where there are gorges so deep that the sun's rays never penetrate to their floors, lies the valley of Hunza. Its crystal-clear waters are fed by glaciers. Its mountain air is clear and unpolluted. And its people are renowned for their longevity. This romantic and remote region was the inspiration for the earthly paradise of Shangri-La in James Hilton's novel *Lost Horizon*.

Hidden in the valley, so it is said, lies the Fountain of Eternal Youth. And the claim has been made that some of the Hunza people have lived to be more than 140 years old, maintaining their vigor almost to the end. We would not expect accurate records to have been kept by a community isolated for centuries behind a barrier of some of the highest mountains in the world, but it seems beyond doubt that the Hunza live to a very ripe old age indeed. Their low-fat diet and their hard-working way of life appear to be part of the secret. At these high altitudes, great effort is needed to grow the rice, corn, apricots, apples, peaches, mulberries, and pears on which they live. Meat is a rarity, and the only oil they use is obtained from apricot kernels. Their very isolation breeds a sense of serenity in which life moves at the rhythm of the seasons and revolves around the raising of crops. Water, of course, is essential. The worst crime of all in the code of the Hunza is not murder but stealing another man's water.

Half a world away, to the West, South America has its own version of Shangri-La—the sub-tropical valley of Vilcabamba in the foothills of the Ecuadorian Andes. Here again, hard work from an early age is accepted as a fact of life, the diet is practically meat free, and the inhabitants have a remarkably high life expectancy. Some, it is claimed, have lived to beyond 130. Whether that claim can be authenticated or not, Vilcabambans are noted for their longevity and for their high resistance to many of the diseases that afflict people in more "advanced" societies—cancer, diabetes, heart disease, rheumatism, and osteoporosis. In the twentieth century they became the subjects of intensive study by leading gerontologists from the U.S.A., Europe, and Japan. The valley produces an abundance of grains, fruit, and vegetables, and its waters are rich in magnesium and other minerals. Most of the visiting scientists agreed that hard work and a healthy diet were the prime factors in the ability of the Vilcabambans to defy old age.

In the matriarchal societies of Italy and Greece, however, it is still not uncommon for sons in their forties to be living at home with other members of the family, joining them at Mama's every Sunday for lunch. Nor is it uncommon for Europeans living in North America.

In such societies, the traditional attitude is not a begrudging one of "having to take care of the parents." Rather, the elders are seen as a source of wisdom and mediation in family quarrels. They are the ones who must be informed, consulted, and obeyed—or at least listened to. In societies that take this role away from the elderly—and sadly our own society seems to have taken this route—it is downhill from then on for the old folks. Stacey Fallon, a social worker in a U.S. retirement home, made a key observation: "We were taking care of them instead of showing them how to take care of themselves."

Many regions of the world lay claim to astonishingly long-living communities. Among them are villages in the Caucasus region of the former Soviet Union, Campodimele in southern Italy, the village of Arachova near Delphi, and the island of Crete. In general, the claims to extreme venerability are not backed by accurate records. This is not so, however, on the Japanese island of Okinawa, where births and deaths have been meticulously recorded in family registers since 1879. The Japanese seem to live longer than anyone else, and Okinawans live longer than other Japanese.

The Japanese Formula for Preventing Damage...

Okinawa has 457 living centenarians—nearly 35 for every 100,000 of the population. The average life expectancy in Okinawa is the longest in the world: eighty-six for women and seventy-eight for men. Their secret, described in a book on the Okinawan centenarians by Bradley and Craig Wilcox and Makoto Suzuki, is a diet rich in vegetables and fruits, soy products, and omega-3 rich fish, along with a good dose of local rice wine. Many of them are farmers and fishermen, so they get plenty of gravity-defying exercise in their daily lives.

The community is imbued with a "help your neighbor" ethic. There is an Okinawan proverb that says, "Once we meet and talk, we are brothers and sisters." One example of the value of this approach came when the Okinawans applied it to solve a serious community problem and at the same time reduce the stress of loneliness and helplessness among the elderly. They were running out of space for a childcare facility and decided to house it in a nursing home for old people. The staff gave childcare assignments to those residents who could manage them, and the results were outstanding.

The youngsters benefited from the extra attention and loving care they were given. The elders found an audience that needed them and gave them a purpose in life. They had something to wake up for, anticipating their meetings with the children and knowing they would be needed again the next day. Even those residents who at first could not handle assignments improved. They were not to be left out. And the dual use of the facility saved money all around. This type of practice is spreading in Japan now. Pen-pal programs with the very elderly, where young children are paired with seniors, are now being used as part of their care. This has the added benefit of teaching young children about the importance of caring for their elders.

...and Their Formula for Harnessing Gravity

For the Japanese, exercise is a way of life and is connected to their reverence for nature, elders, and ancestors. They walk a lot. Their brand of exercise, not unlike Chinese *tai chi*, consists of slow, precise, controlled movements requiring exceptional balance and mental concentration. Though rapidly disappearing, their lifestyle of eating and sleeping on *tatami* mats, which lie directly on the floor, includes a great deal of knee bending, posture change, and squatting. This is a perfect formula for harnessing gravity. It stimulates the vestibular gravity receptors of the inner ear, tunes blood-pressure reflexes, and uses the body's own weight to load muscles and bones.

The Negative Impact of Modern Lifestyles

The most convincing evidence for the benefits of this lifestyle came from data on 100,000 Okinawans who moved to Brazil in the early twentieth century and adopted the dietary habits of their new home. Despite good genes, their life expectancy was shortened by seventeen years compared to those who stayed back home. Even in Okinawa, those under fifty who have grown up with fast-food outlets surrounding the U.S. military bases now have Japan's highest rates of obesity, heart disease, and premature death.

Where Women Have the Edge...

All over the world, women outlive men. Japanese women have the world's longest lifespan, at 83.9 years, compared to 77.3 years for their men folk. Spanish women come a close second, with a life expectancy of 82.7 years, the longest in Europe. At the other end of the scale, the women of Sierra Leone in West Africa have the shortest lifespan, at 39.8 years. Men in Sierra Leone live on average for 35.9 years. U.S. women rank fifteenth in life expectancy, at eighty years. Because men die younger, 70% of nursing-home occupants in the U.S.A. are women.

What is the secret of women's greater longevity? If we could discover it, could we use it to extend the lives of men? Understanding the reasons for this gender difference in longevity is a goldmine that remains to be tapped. We are just starting to recognize that gender does matter in a lot of clinical conditions. There are differences between men and women in every system of the body, right down to how nutrients and drugs are absorbed, metabolized, and ultimately used by the body.

Women seem to have developed better coping skills, not least through their greater reliance on support groups. In general, they need more social interaction and are more communicative about their emotions than men. Managing stress and communicating with others appear to be aspects of life where women have an advantage. They are more likely to seek help, to make and keep friends, to take care of sick parents or grandchildren, and to volunteer to care for others. In essence, they never stop working, and that may be the secret of their longevity.

...and Where Women Miss Out

Women may live longer than men, but in many ways their lives are harder. Working women have always had to take care of a home and family as well as go to their outside jobs. Those who have been kept in the dark about family finances and sheltered by their husbands from decision making are more likely to deteriorate when the husband or partner dies. They lose the sense that they are needed. If they are lucky, they will regard this as the opportunity for a new start.

Lenore Brown, a former geriatric nurse at Holly Manor, Mendham, New Jersey, tells the story of a couple in their nineties who were in the nursing home. The wife doted on her husband, making quite sure the staff attended to his every need. She would not leave his company. The couple took their meals in their own room, facing each other. Then, at ninety-two, the husband died. A few days later, the staff was amazed to see his widow come with her walker down the hall and ask, "Which way is the bingo game?"

Many an older woman suddenly finding herself alone does not emerge as such a self-sufficient, independent individual. They may go into rapid decline, and even the effort of shopping or cooking for one may seem pointless and overwhelming. Single women who have had to fend for themselves all their lives and have developed their own circle of friends have an advantage in later life. This was confirmed by the MacArthur Successful Aging Study of the eighties, which found that older single people of both sexes, but women in particular, had indeed sharper minds than their married counterparts.

Women are not only the most numerous among the elderly, they are also the poorest. Their pensions are lower than those of men, because most worked at lower paying jobs and their careers were often part time or fragmented for family reasons. A woman who has never worked may find that her benefits are halved when the man dies, though her outgoings remain much the same.

The Male Advantage

At every stage of life, men are more vulnerable to premature death. But once past the danger zone of forty-five to sixty-five, their life expectancy increases and the gender gap narrows. A man of seventy in the U.S. can expect to see at least his eighty-second birthday, as compared to eighty-five for his female counterpart. Men who live to a hundred tend to have been self-employed, and rarely have they taken early retirement. Men over ninety, in general, function better mentally and physically than women of the same age. This is probably because they have been and continue to be more physically and mentally active.

The Retirement Years

The traditional retirement gift is a watch or a clock. It is kindly meant, but perhaps it also symbolizes the subconscious thought that the recipient's real life is over; all he or she can now do is count the days and wait to die. In fact, it is not unusual to hear stories of people who do die within a couple of years of retirement. It seems to make no difference whether stopping work was mandatory or happened as the result of family pressure. Those who age successfully point to the importance of actively planning for retirement, including the pursuit of many interests and passions. This forward thinking is mostly started long before the dreaded date of parting from the structured life of daily office or factory work.

Astronauts Who Simply Refuse to "Fade Away"

Careful preparation and planning become second nature to the kind of human beings who are prepared to climb aboard a tiny capsule on top of a rocket thirty-six stories high that can develop up to 7 million pounds of thrust and blast them into the void. John Glenn took up politics after his first trip into space and became a U.S. senator. So did Harrison "Jack" Schmidt, who in 1972 piloted *Apollo 17* to the Moon. John Sweigert, who flew on *Apollo 13* on the abortive mission to the Moon, was elected to Congress in 1982 but died before taking his seat. Neil Armstrong, the first man to set foot on the Moon, became a professor of Aeronautical Engineering at the University of Cincinnati. Buzz Aldrin, who followed him on to the Moon, is an inventor, writer, speaker, and product-endorser in television commercials. Alan Shepard, the first American to fly in space and the man who hit a golf ball on the Moon, served as director on the boards of several companies, including the Coors Brewing Company. Charles "Pete" Conrad, who flew on the early Gemini missions, ended up as vice president of a cable TV firm and became a consultant on the development of space rides for Walt Disney.

They and many other astronauts followed in the American tradition of self-help. The Soviet cosmonauts, on the other hand, were looked after by the state when they "retired" from space. They became national heroes, celebrities who were rewarded with *dachas*—luxurious country homes—and paid to tour the country, giving inspiring lectures to schoolchildren.

If You Don't Have a Dream...

Looking forward instead of dwelling on the past is essential to a positive attitude towards aging. If you do not have something to look forward to, you will probably have a hard time getting up in the morning. In far too many nursing homes, the residents find that yesterday, today, and tomorrow all blur into the same monotonous routine of peering at some talking head on the TV screen. The staff however well meaning, do not help if they treat the residents like patients or children.

When I first started doing bed-rest studies at NASA, I noticed that the very healthy young men who volunteered quickly started behaving like patients in a hospital. The staff, used to caring only for the sick lying in bed, treated them as such. If asked how they felt, the volunteers responded with a tirade that listed all their childhood illnesses—chicken pox, measles, and all.

This was hardly the way to foster a positive attitude, so we quickly took action to remove all possible trappings and behaviors associated with hospitals. White lab coats were replaced by colorful aprons. Staff no longer wore stethoscopes around their necks, and they were trained and constantly reminded that these volunteers were healthier than they themselves were. If you apply the lessons learned from this experience to a nursing-home environment, you can see not only how easily minor discomforts take on overwhelming proportions, but also how the hopelessness and resignation that come with being treated like a patient can be countered.

When It Comes to Retirement, Failing to Plan Is Planning to Fail

Those who are lucky enough to work at an art or craft or science never really retire in the sense that they never stop doing the job they love, though they may change the conditions under which they pursue it. Professional people, such as doctors or nurses, accountants or teachers, can turn to voluntary work. Most people, however, just do not know what to do with themselves after they have retired. They can quickly feel despair and depression. The jobs around the house they had been able to avoid because of work become an unavoidable burden. If pension or social security have removed the financial incentive for continuing to work, if the children are now grown up and do not need you, and if all your life the *job* directed what you did, where now is your motivation to get up and do something?

Travel may provide some temporary relief. You may take a course, but your heart is not in it. You have not engaged in sport for years, except to watch it on TV. Your job was your life, and your friends were all work colleagues who within a year or so have become more distant. Your wife, after making a short effort to do things with you, goes back to her interests and friends. Every time she goes to her exercise class or her bridge game, you become more despondent. You bring down your toy train set from the attic, but after the second day the magic is gone. So you numb your helplessness with beer, pretzels, potato chips, and TV, or you sit in front of your computer. You forward reams of jokes to a list of people, most of whom you do not know. You play solitaire and surf the web looking for something that can give you an answer to your dilemma. To be brutally honest, you are waiting to die. It may be that women live longer because they adjust more easily to retirement. However, as they move up on the career scale separation from the workplace may have similar consequences to that most often seen in men.

The good news is that life in retirement need not be like this. All it takes is some early post-retirement career planning. Just like putting away money for retirement is not achieved overnight, so the mental adjustment to a change in routine, responsibilities, and social interactions—including more time with your spouse—takes time to happen.

The Economic Imperative

Money is not everything, but the state of your health and your capacity to enjoy the later years can depend on the state of your wallet. The current trend of people living longer and the likelihood that life spans will increase even further over the next fifty years have generated alarm among economists and politicians. How can the population still at work support and provide medical care for this mushrooming segment of pensioners?

Julia Alvarez, poet and UN Ambassador at large from the Dominican Republic, calls it the "agequake" or "age wave," and it has become a matter of worldwide concern. In 2021, the first of the USA's 76 million baby boomers will turn seventy-five.

The Pensions Dilemma

Extending working life so that more people contribute to the economy, rather than only drawing from the Treasury, could be an important way of lightening the burden on the shrinking workforce. Otherwise, they will have to carry the increasing cost of supporting the mushrooming older population for forty or fifty years beyond retirement. A potential backlash or rebellion of the workforce may well result when they discover they can no longer bear the financial and emotional load of these costs. However, politicians know that asking the working population to wait longer to draw their pensions would be a deeply unpopular move. In any case, with the highest fertility rate in the developed world, the U.S. may be in a better position to handle the problem of a shrinking workforce than many countries.

Japan appears to be less fortunate. A projection released by the country's National Institute of Population and Social Security Research predicts a decline in the number of children at the same time as an increase in the number of the elderly. The population of Japan, now 120 million, is projected to peak in 2006 at 127.74 million. By 2050, if present trends continue, 37.5% of the Japanese population will be over sixty-five, compared with 17.4% in 2000. It is not difficult to see that a drastic overhaul is needed in pension and medical care systems, which have been built on assumptions that no longer hold true.

Many countries have tested pension reforms, but most, as in Japan for instance, have been based strictly on economics—cutting benefits and raising contributions—without factoring in the well-being of the individual. In 2004, the center-right French government of Prime Minister Jean-Pierre Raffarin suffered a humiliating defeat in regional elections on just this issue.

Swedish reform measures link retirement benefits both to contributions and to life expectancy. The earlier one retires after sixty-one, the lower the benefit; the longer one continues working, the higher the benefit. Swedes can also take a portion of their retirement benefit while working part time. Other European countries are looking into adapting the Swedish system to their own needs.

To Enjoy a Good Life, Keep on Working—and It Hardly Matters at What

Economics aside, there are very good psychological and health reasons for extending working life. The work need not be paid work: being productive, staying busy, and feeling needed are major positive factors in remaining healthy and independent. The issue of when we should retire will continue to cause problems if it is only based on some arbitrary chronological age, for "real age" is not the same for everybody.

Suitable incentives should be provided for both employers and employees to motivate people to extend their working lives, albeit possibly not in the same job nor at full pay. Insurance companies could be encouraged to provide such incentives in the form of discounted premiums for people who remain earners longer. Just as the discounts for not smoking have done their part to save many lives, premium reductions for staying lean and active would benefit both individuals and society. Incentives might be designed to take advantage of what we have learned from space about the deleterious effects of inactivity and the dramatic benefits of using the gravity in which we live.

The Case for an *Elder Corps*

In the days when most jobs were physically demanding and far from emotionally satisfying, many people looked forward to retirement, and a set retirement age was necessary. It also made way for women and the younger generation to move into the workforce. But today, that workforce is shrinking, and there seem to be only three solutions: export jobs, import workers, or extend the working life.

Instead of delaying Social Security to some later age, perhaps it could be phased in over a period of five, ten, or even fifteen years. A homeland Elder Corps could be established, rather like the Peace Corps, which now attracts mostly younger people. The skills of fifty to eighty-year-olds could be matched against a "needs inventory" for community-related jobs. This work would be paid, to supplement their social security. At present, we have in America a host of community needs which, when left to unpaid volunteers, are not always successfully met. An Elder Corps could draw on people with proven skills in administration, education, mentoring, technical writing and consulting, career counseling, the care of children and older olds, medical and scientific support, home care, transportation and security, publishing, advertising, and the arts.

The Retired and Senior Volunteer Program (RSVP), which has been around for thirty years, already places older persons as volunteers in schools, museums, hospitals, and a host of other organizations. It works well, but my own experience with other volunteer organizations is that some of them are not interested in older people and that they can be unfriendly and discouraging. Volunteers are sometimes put off after finding that paid employees of the organization may not bother to explore and make use of the volunteers' particular skills and talents. It is generally thought of as women's work, because it is mostly service oriented. In many instances, those who do not volunteer are the very ones who should be encouraged to do so, because they are the ones who most need to become physically, socially, and mentally active to regain their self-worth and remain healthy.

Under the Elder Corps scheme, workers would be managed by their peers, given responsibility, made accountable, and given the economic incentive to remain active and independent. Employers would have the incentive of retaining or hiring skilled and experienced workers at a lower cost, since salaries would be subsidized by their pension or Social Security.

When he first became Britain's Prime Minister in 1940, early in World War II, Winston Churchill was sixty-six and was thought of as an old man. In a recent splendid biography, Roy Jenkins pointed out, "The comment that Churchill is aging (beyond the routine ticking of the chronological clock) was frequent at the time, but there was remarkably little support for it in the output of his working day, and there is strong suspicion more of wishful thinking than of hard evidence." In 1954, when he was eighty years old and again at the helm as Prime Minister, he held a luncheon where guests included Osbert Peake, the Minister of Pensions and National Insurance, the equivalent of our Social Security Administration. Churchill wrote, "Peake hates old people (as such) living too long and cast a critical eye at me. He told about his father, who was stone blind for twenty years and kept alive at great expense by three nurses till he died reluctantly at ninety-one, and of course the Death Duties were ever so much more than they would have been if he had only been put out of the way earlier. I felt very guilty. But in rejoinder I took him into my study and showed him the four packets of proofs of the *History of the English Speaking Peoples*, which bring 50,000 dollars a year into this island on my account alone. 'You don't keep me, I keep you.' He was rather taken aback."

The Secrets of Healthy Aging

The Chicago-based MacArthur Foundation funded research in the 1980s that allowed sixteen scientists to study the physical and mental health of 1,189 people in their seventies over a period of ten years. When asked their secret, those who were aging successfully frequently replied, "Just keep on going." The scientists concluded, "It is this forward-looking, active engagement with life and with other human beings that is so critical to growing old well."

Sporting Life and Sporting Legends

More and more elderly people are working out in the gym these days, and there are special classes for those once thought too delicate and frail to exercise. It is no longer rare to see runners, cyclists and, of course, golfers who are well over seventy. In 2001, at the age of 101, Harold Stilson of Boca Raton, Florida, set the record for the oldest golfer to score a hole-in-one on the 108-yard par-three sixteenth hole of the Deerfield Country Club in Deerfield Beach, Florida. Stilson, who has a 27 handicap, drives to the course to play eighteen holes three times a week.

Golfers stay young to a ripe old age. All over the United States, retirement communities are springing up around golf courses. The high handicappers simply enjoy the game, while the star players can add good prize money to the pleasure they get from the competition and from hitting the ball where it is intended to go. Legendary figures such as Jack Nicklaus, Tom Watson, Hale Irwin, and South African Gary Player are all regular entrants in the over-fifties Champions Tour. In 2002, at the age of fifty-five, Bruce Fleisher totaled $1.8 million in prize money. At seventy-four, Arnie Palmer competed (by invitation) in the 2004 Masters Tournament, in Augusta, Georgia.

Paul Newman, now seventy-nine, still enjoys getting into the cockpit of a racing car and driving it round the circuit. John Glenn, eighty-three years old in 2004, flies his airplane between Ohio and Washington, D.C. Mabel Birkner, a celebrated big-game hunter, took to the field at the age of one hundred at the start of the deer season. President Gerald Ford, who played football for the University of Michigan and now keeps fit with regular golf, celebrated his ninety-first birthday in 2004 and is as sharp as ever. Ann Boyle Gallagher of Alexandria, Virginia, skydived for the first time at seventy-eight. When asked why, she said it was on her list of things she had not yet done. President George H. W. Bush celebrated his eightieth birthday in June 2004 by parachuting twice 13,000 ft out of a plane, only to be outdone by 101-year-old Australian Frank Moody, who did it on a bet. Bush's message to his contemporaries, "Get out and do something. Don't just sit around watching TV."

Markets are changing to meet this new sports sector. The Senior Olympics in the U.S. and the European Veterans' Athletics Championships provide grueling competition. The United States Tennis Association now has an over-nineties tennis league. In 1999, Emil Johnson of Orlando, Florida, won the national men's over-ninety division and at ninety-two was named U.S. Tennis Association Florida's Player of the Year. Dorothy "Dodo" Cheney, now eighty-eight, is tennis's most decorated champion, having won 312 USTA championships. May Sutton Bundy, Dodo's mother, won the Wimbledon championship in 1905—the first American to do so—and kept playing tennis into her early eighties as well. What keeps such people going? Dodo says, "Competition. Keep doing it...play through your injuries...don't stop."

Fauja Singh, a ninety-three-year-old Sikh, ran the 2004 London marathon, completing the 26-mile 385-yard run in 6 hrs 7 min. It was his seventh marathon since coming to England from the Punjab eleven years ago. Fauja, who lives in Redbridge, Essex, was an athlete in his youth who returned to running as a form of therapy after his son was killed in a road accident. He is a whippet-thin non-smoking, non-drinking vegetarian who meditates every morning and prays every day. His time in 2004 was only four minutes longer than in 2003. His bone density is apparently that of a fifty-year-old. He is living proof that there is no such thing as being too old.

Soon after Fauja's success, one-hundred-year-old Philip Rabinowitz, from Cape Town, South Africa, broke the 100-m dash record for centenarians, at 30.86 seconds. As if that were not enough, he had to run again because the clock had failed the first time! His secret to a long, healthy life: fresh orange juice before breakfast and an apple after each meal. He recommends moderation, work, and walking. Many over sixty-five would be glad to match his time.

High-performance athletes never cease to impress. Lucille Bergen amazed the crowd by winning the women's National Water Ski championship in the slalom and tricks event. An achievement in itself, it was even more noteworthy because the event took place on her ninety-first birthday, on August 9, 2004.

Do What You Love Doing

Poet Laureate Stanley Kunitz, born 1905, put it this way: "What makes the engine go? Desire, desire, desire." People with a craft they love can continue to practice their skills and exercise the brain and soul as long as they live. And for this reason they live longer and longer.

Good scientists fall into that category. They retain youthful curiosity, solving nature's jigsaw puzzle and trying to imagine how things work. At 102, Dr. Ray Crist is a visiting professor of Environmental Science at the Kline Hall of Science at Messiah College, in Pennsylvania. His research on the effects of toxic materials on the environment is still a "hot" topic. As he puts it, "I just do it. I don't think about it. I don't have sense enough to quit."

Hold On to Your Zest for Life

Patience and persistence are part and parcel of daily political life and may explain the longevity and "never-say-die" spirit of some politicians. Senator Strom Thurmond (R-SC), born in 1902, retired from the Senate in 2002 after celebrating his one hundredth birthday. He died shortly after that. Another remarkable example of political endurance was the British MP Emmanuel "Manny" Shinwell (1884–1986), a fiery Scot first elected to Parliament in 1931 who rode the bus to the Houses of Parliament even at the age of one hundred. In debate he became Churchill's favorite sparring partner. In due course, this feisty man became known as "Father of the House."

Great Britain's beloved Queen Mum, Queen Elizabeth the Queen Mother, who died in 2001 at the age of 101, was a splendid example of irrepressible *joie de vivre.* Like so many active centenarians, she enjoyed a drink—in her case, good wine or a gin and Dubonnet. She underwent a hip operation, but after receiving a blood transfusion on her one-hundredth birthday, she headed off for a four-and-a-half-hour visit to the Royal Ballet at Covent Garden. No one dared to suggest to this fiercely determined woman that it was time to take things easy.

France's Marie Brémont (1886–2002) died at 116. When she turned 100 years of age, she still walked five miles daily to do her shopping, declining offers of a lift and proclaiming, "Walking is what keeps me healthy!" Age did not suppress her coquetry. She liked red, which flattered her complexion, and had a hairdresser do her hair regularly. Her secret for longevity? "I have always been happy."

In 2002, I encountered a group of impressive women, all of them either former winners of the Ms. Virginia Senior America title or interested in becoming contestants. What struck me about these women was their philosophy on life. They had all suffered some debilitating hardship and had entered the competition in order to prod themselves back into an active lifestyle.

One of them, sixty-seven-year-old Jane Lytle, summarized their approach to aging as follows: "The cardinal rule is to keep your calendar full. Look forward, don't be afraid to have a dream, and when you do, share it with others. God gave you the gift of life. Treat it well, take time to forgive, share moments, dream, and especially laugh. Climb high and far and reach for the stars. Life is not static. Make adjustments and you will live a full life. Live life as an adventure." She went on, "Prior to the pageant, age was a number, and mine was unlisted, but now I seize this moment in time, for it will not pass my way again. Seize this moment to praise, smile. Aging is not the end but the beginning. Start by giving your best and the best will come back to you. This is our age of elegance. Share a smile. Accentuate the positive."

Be a Child Again

If you want to be reminded of what you need to do to get the best out of gravity, think back to when you were a child. You can learn much by watching a baby use gravity unconsciously as it develops. Holding its head up, pushing up on its hands, rolling over, learning how to stand—first with its feet wide apart like an astronaut returning from space or an old person trying to keep their balance—a baby is coming to terms with gravity.

Gradually the baby will move its feet closer and closer together and then lift its feet and plant them down firmly when it walks, and next thing you know, that baby is a toddler and is running. Then come games of hop-scotch and cartwheels and handstands and swings, with gravity stimulating the inner ear and different parts of the body. Whistling, yelling, and singing that stimulate the facial muscles. Next they engage in sport of some kind. And never forget the curiosity and sense of wonder that play such a key role in the lives of children.

The college years bring more intellectual pursuits. Work, family, and responsibilities follow. As the stresses of life multiply, bad habits creep in. Stop using gravity effectively and disabilities move in, no matter what your age. What you become at fifty, sixty, seventy, or a hundred depends on what you do at twenty, thirty, forty, and onwards.

Building Up Reserves

Astronauts clearly have a head start in terms of fitness because of their training and because they are hand picked for it in the first place. They are fully aware of the bodily and mental changes brought about by that much-coveted stay in space. They are therefore very conscientious about building up their reserves before they are launched. An excellent example of this is the increase in bone density they achieve as a result of their well-rounded exercise program before their flight. The bones in the lower half of their bodies can be as much as 30% denser and therefore stronger than if they had only been generally active. They still lose a great deal of bone in space. But even after a flight, their bone density can be within the normal range for their age.

The connection between space and aging is gravity. Gravity's value is diminished on earth through our own increasing inactivity. The result: same changes as in space but developing over a much longer time—a lifetime.

The active old have resisted the temptation to give in to such habits. What you see in them is the result of a lifetime of good habits: a sensible diet, effective stress management, and, whether they are aware of it or not, the right approach to harnessing gravity.

They do not dwell on problems. They have a positive, forward-looking attitude and plenty of social and intellectual stimulation. They have a good sense of humor. They follow a life of routine and structure. This helps them sleep well at night. They are up and about during the day, doing some form of work, because they really have never stopped working, even though they may not be doing the job they did for most of their lives and may not be getting paid for it. Their reward is that they enjoy every single minute of their lives.

The "Magic Cure" Is in Your Hands

We live in an age of sound bites and quick fixes. TV commercials must put their message across in less than a minute if they are to catch and hold our attention. Books and magazines promise quick weight loss, a sculpted body, or a wrinkle-free face—all achieved with no pain or sweat and usually in a few weeks. Yet most are hard to stick with. They are either impractical, take too much time, or just don't fulfill their promises. Believe me, I have tried most of them! The reason? We try to hoodwink Mother Nature, always looking for the shortcut.

I am often told that people will not make a long-term commitment to alter their lifestyles for the sake of better health. The constant refrain is "Tell me what pill, herb, or nutritional supplement I can take to fix everything." Drug discoveries have done wonders in treating damage from disease and reducing some health risks. But there is no universal pill to keep us young or to keep most diseases at bay. Insofar as there is a "magic" cure to many of the problems associated with age, it lies within us. We hold the key to the box with the magic cure.

Inside this box is a lifetime plan of accumulating good habits. We start off with an overall assessment of where we are, setting goals for where we would like to be and how much time and effort we are willing to invest in staying young. It is our life-insurance policy, except that we are the beneficiaries, rewarded with an active and independent life.

- **Step one** of the action plan is preventing whatever damage and ceasing whatever damaging habits we have collected along the way. No quick fix, or even slow program, has a chance of working unless we manage what we eat and drink and learn how to cope effectively with stress. Everyone makes mistakes in life, but it is a bit like the board game of Snakes and Ladders. After sliding down a snake, you cannot make progress until you climb up a ladder again.

- **Step two** is becoming informed, learning, and thinking about gravity. You need to understand how gravity affects your body. How and when can you use it? What can you do to draw on this powerful stimulus more often or more efficiently? Outline a series of habits you want to acquire over a period of time to fulfill your goals. How will you measure success?

- **Step three** is taking action in a slow and systematic way to build up a reserve of good habits. Diversify your portfolio of activities to add variety so that even if you have to give up one or two activities for a time, you can press ahead with the others. Keep the engine tuned and the support structures loaded.

A Book for the Young

Good planning starts early, whether the goal is secure finances or good health. You have probably heard of stories of old folks ending up in nursing homes. You may not be aware of the many energetic, active, and independent people of the same age and their surprising achievements. They are already practicing the methods laid out in this book, even though they may not be aware of the whys and wherefores.

Although it is never too late to start using gravity properly, the fact remains that those who start early in life are doing themselves a great favor. My message should be of special value to the young, who have the opportunity to choose their outcome and who want to be able to carry on enjoying life when they are ready to retire. You may well be investing during your working years in a long-term financial retirement plan to provide you with adequate financial resources. You can hardly wait to travel and discover all those places you never seemed to have the time to visit while you worked. But you may find that at this crucial stage in your life you no longer have the stamina and health resources to enjoy life to the full. To avoid arriving at this impasse, you need to start investing in yourself, now. Acquire gravity-using habits to build up your bodily reserves so that you remain young and vigorous in those later years.

Epilogue

Lessons from Space

The previous chapters set out on a surprising journey of discovery, tracing a line from astronauts to gravity to aging. They challenge the widely held belief that certain changes that come with aging are unavoidable. Yes, the theory is provocative. But research in space and on Earth in support of the astronauts have shown convincingly that adopting a lifestyle that uses gravity less and less over many years lies at the root of the early signs of what we call *aging*.

This research has taught us two things. First, age in years is not always linked to the physical and mental changes that we have come to associate with someone who is *old*, from thinning bones to failing memory. These changes can take place at almost any age. Astronauts in space experience them, and they are hardly old. Healthy college student volunteers lying in bed for weeks also experience them. Even children are not exempt. Type-2 diabetes (the type associated with being inactive and overweight), high blood pressure, and clogged arteries all used to be more or less confined to people over fifty but are now showing up in children.

Secondly, changes often blamed on "getting old" can be delayed or reversed whatever our age. They are readily reversible in astronauts and bed-rest volunteers when they once more begin to move about in Earth's gravity. Research has shown that light training with weights can restore lost muscle mass and bone density and strengthen muscle and bone even in ninety-year-olds. Imagine how much more effective the tailored use of gravity would be in those who are much younger.

Redefining Aging

Aging is simply the passing of time. It was once believed to follow the end of reproductive activity, much like senescent cells in the body that stop dividing but still live on. But there seems to be no natural limit to man's reproductive potency, and menopause in women in the Western world occurs later than it used to.

I believe that the signs of aging often become most evident whenever growth and development stops. In fact, aging starts even earlier. Cells die as new ones are formed even in the developing embryo. But when an individual is growing and developing, the new cells outpace those that are lost. The reverse happens when growth stops. New cells are still created, but more are lost. This phase is now considered to start around the age of twenty-five. Few today would think of people in their thirties as old despite the odd gray hair or the appearance of a first wrinkle.

Your state of health and fitness at your peak, reached at the end of the growth phase, is therefore crucial. It may be bone strength, brain development, or any of the myriad other factors that enable us to function. This peak level establishes the rate at which bone may be lost or problems such as poor balance may emerge.

The rate of decline that inevitably follows the end of the growth period depends on our lifestyle habits. In some, like the remarkable Fauja Singh who ran the marathon at ninety-three and whose bones are said to be those of someone forty years his junior, the decline may be almost imperceptible. In others, the downward slope may be very steep. At a much younger age, it brings with it wasting muscles and bones, unsteady walking, and the host of reversible changes we have seen in astronauts returning from space.

How steep the slope will be and at what age the first signs of aging will appear are the direct results of the care we take to prevent damage and harness gravity. Maintaining the habits and activities that challenge gravity and that stood us well during development should continue to keep us young in body and spirit for a long time.

We know that the changes associated with the passage of time, whether slow or comparatively rapid in their onset, are not universal. Not everyone develops balance problems or a sudden drop in blood pressure on standing. Not everyone suffers the ravages of osteoporosis, disturbed sleep, and memory loss.

What does harnessing gravity mean? You automatically harness gravity any time you make a movement. It is important to make yourself aware of when you are using gravity most during your day's activities and when you are not. Check the amount of time you spend each day performing tasks that do not harness gravity and increase the amount of time and ways in which you do. Make this a habit. Catch yourself when you slip up and make up for lost time as soon as you can. Essentially, think about what you want to be able to do in later years, and just keep doing it throughout your life. Once you understand the connection of what you do in everyday life with gravity, you are well on your way to success.

No one can halt the passage of time. But some people stand out as independent, energetic, and full of life. They look and act fifteen years younger than others of the same age. By adopting a lifestyle that consciously and deliberately harnesses gravity, you can reverse or delay the changes that come with what the world calls *aging*.

Selected Bibliography and Resources

Chapter 1

Dietrick, J. E., G. D. Whedon, E. Shorr, V. Toscani, V. B. Davis. "Effect of Immobilization on Metabolic and Physiologic Functions of Normal Men." *American Journal of Medicine* 4 (1948): 3–35.

Nicogossian, A. E., C. L. Huntoon, S. L. Poole. *Space Physiology and Medicine*, Philadelphia: Lea and Febiger, 1994.

Sandler, H, J. Vernikos. (Editors) *Inactivity: Physiological Effects*, New York: Academic Press, Inc., 1986

Vernikos, J. "Human Physiology in Space." *BioEssays* 18 (1996): 1029-1037.

Chapter 2

Bekker, P. J., D. Holloway, A. Nakashini, M. Arrighi, P. T. Leese, C. R. Dunstan. "The Effect of a Single Dose of Osteoprotegerin in Postmenopausal Women." *Journal of Bone and Mineral Research* 16 (2001): 348-360.

Cardinale, M., C. Bosco. "The Effects of Vibration as an Exercise Intervention." *Exercise & Sport Sciences Reviews* 31 (2003): 3-7.

Morey Holton, E. R., R. T. Whalen, S. B. Arnaud, M. C. Van Der Meulen. "The Skeleton and its Adaptation to Gravity," In: *Handbook of Physiology, Section 4: Environmental Physiology* (M.J.Fregly and C.M.Blatteis, Eds.) New York: Oxford University Press, Volume 1 (1996): 691-720.

New, S. A., S. P. Robins, J. C. Martin, M. J. Garton, C. Bolton-Smith, D. A.Grubb, S. J. Lee, D. M. Reid. "Dietary Influence on Bone Mass and Bone Metabolism—Further Evidence of a Positive Link Between Fruit and

Vegetable Consumption and Bone Health?" *American Journal of Clinical Nutrition* 71 (2000): 142-151.

Rubin, C., G. Xu, S. Judex. "The Anabolic Activity of Bone Tissue, Suppressed by Disuse, is Normalized by Brief Exposure to Extremely Low-magnitude Mechanical Stimuli". *Federation of American Societies for Experimental Biology Journal* 15 (2001): 2225-2229.

Rubin, C., A. S. Turner, S. Bain, C. Mallinckrodt, K. McLeod. "Anabolism. Low Mechanical Signals Strengthen Long Bones." *Nature* 412 (2001): 603-604.

Rubin, C., A. S. Turner, C. Mallinckrodt, C. Jerome, K. McLeod, S. Bain. "Mechanical Strain, Induced Non-invasively in the High Frequency Domain, is Anabolic to Cancellous Bone, but Not Cortical Bone." *Bone* 30 (2002): 445-452.

Turner, R. T. "Physiology of Microgravity Environment: What we know about the Effects of Spaceflight on Bone?" *Journal of Applied Physiology* 89 (2000): 840-847.

Chapter 3

Adams, G. R., V. J. Caiozzo, K. M. Baldwin. "Skeletal Muscle Unweighting: Spaceflight and Ground-based Models." *Journal of Applied Physiology* 95 (2000): 2185-2201.

Booth, F. W., S. E. Gordon, C. J. Carlson, M. T. Hamilton. "Waging War on Modern Chronic Diseases: Primary Prevention through Exercise Biology." *Journal of Applied Physiology* 88 (2000): 774-787.

Booth, F. W., M. V. Chakravarthy, E. E. Sangenberg. "Exercise and Gene Expression: Physiological Regulation of the Human Genome through Physical Activity." *Journal of Physiology (London)* 543 (2002): 399-411.

Chakravarthy, M. V., F. W. Booth. "Eating, Exercise, and 'Thrifty' Genotypes: Connecting the Dots toward an Evolutionary Understanding of Modern Chronic Diseases." *Journal of Appied Physiology* 96 (2004): 3-10.

Evans, W. J., G. S. Couzens. *AstroFit.* New York: The Free Press, 2002.

Lee, S. M. C., J. M. Loehr, D. Nguyen, S. M. Schneider. "Foot-Ground Reaction Force during Resistive Exercise in Parabolic Flight." *Aviation Space and Environmental Medicine* 75 (2004): 405-412.

Manson, J. E., F. B. Hu, J. W. Rich-Edwards, G. A. Colditz, M. J. Stampfer, W. C. Willett, F. E. Speizer, C. H. Hennekens. "A Prospective Study of Walking Compared with Vigorous Exercise in the Prevention of Coronary Heart Disease in Women. *New England Journal of Medicine* 341 (1999): 650-658.

Manson, J. E., D. M. Nathan, A. S. Krolewski, M. J. Stampfer, W. C. Willett, C. H. Hennekens. "A Prospective Study of Exercise and Incidence of Diabetes among U.S. Male Physicians." *Journal of American Medical Association* 268 (1992): 63-67.

Wang, E. "Age-dependent Atrophy and Microgravity Travel: What Do They Have In Common?" *Federation of American Societies for Experimental Biology Journal* 13 (1999):S167-S174.

Centers for Disease Control and Prevention. "Self-reported Physical Inactivity by Degree of Urbanization–United States." *Morbidity Mortality Weekly Report* 47 (1998):1097-1100.
www.pilates-studi.com

Chapter 4

Bloomberg, J. J., B. T. Peters, S. L. Smith, W. P. Huebner, M. F. Reschke. "Locomotor Head-trunk Coordination Strategies Following Spaceflight." *Journal of Vestibular Research* 7 (1997): 161-177.

Edgerton, V. R., R. L. deLeon, N. Tillakaratne, M. R. Recktenwal, J. A. Hodgson, R. R. Roy. "Use-dependent Plasticity in Spinal Stepping and Standing." In: *Advances in Neurology: Neuronal Regeneration, Reorganization and Repair,* F.J. Seil (ed.) 72 (1997): 233-248, Philadelphia: Lippincott-Raven Publishers.

Hansen, R., J. Taylor. *Rick Hansen: Man in Motion.* Vancouver: Douglas and McIntyre, 1999.

Jarnlo, G. B. "Hip Fracture Patients: Background and Function." *Scandinavian Journal of Rehabilitation Medicine* 24 (Suppl) (1991): 1-31.

Polaski, W. W. H., M. F. Reschke, F. O. Black, D. D. Doxey, D. L. Harm. "Recovery of Postural Equilibrium Control Following Spaceflight." In: *Sensing and Controlling Motion: Vestibular and Sensorimotor Function.*" B.Cohen, D.L.Tomko and F. Guedry (eds.) New York: New York Academy of Sciences, 1992, pp.747-754.

Province, M. A., F. C. Hadley, M. C. M. C. Hornbrook, L.A. Lipsitz, J.P. Miller, C. D. Mulrow, M. G. Ory, R. W. Sattin, M. E. Tinetti, S. L. Wolf. "The Effects of Exercise on Falls in Elderly Patients. Atlanta FICSIT Group." *Journal American Medical Association* 273(1995): 1341-1347.

Rikli, R., D. J. Edwards. "Effects of a Three-year Exercise Program on Motor Function and Cognitive Processing Speed in Older Women." *Research Quarterly of Exercise and Sport* 62 (1991): 61-67.

Ross, M. D. "A Spaceflight Study of Synaptic Plasticity in Adult Rat Vestibular Maculas." *Acta Oto-Laryngologica* Suppl.516 (1994): 1-14.

Spirduso,W.W. "Aging and Motor Control." In:*Perspectives in Exercise Science and Sports Medicine. Exercise in Older Adults.* C.V.Gisolfi, D.R.Lamb and E.Nadel (eds.), Indiana: Cooper Publishing Group 8 (1995): 53-114.

Tse, S. K., D. M.Bailey. "T'ai Chi and Postural Control in the Well Elderly." *American Journal of Occupational Therapy* 46 (1992): 295-300.

Vestibular Disorders Association: www.vestibular.org; Tel: 1-800-837-8428.

National Institute on Deafness and Other Communication Disorders Information Clearinghouse: www.nidcd.nih.gov. Click on 'Health Information,' then click on 'Hearing & Balance'; Tel: 1-800837-8428.

Johns Hopkins Research and Training Center for Hearing and Balance: www.bme.jhu.edu/labs/chb/index.html or www.bme.jhu.edu/labs/chb/faq.html.

University of Connecticut Health Center–Taste and Smell Center www.uchc.edu/unconntasteandsmell

Chapter 5

Convertino, V. A. "Exercise and Adaptation to Microgravity Environments." In: *Handbook of Physiology, Section 4:Environmental Physiology,* (M.J. Fregly and C.M.Blatteis, Eds.) New York: Oxford University Press, Volume 2 (1996) pp.815-843.

Convertino, V. A., D. F.Doerr, D. L. Eckberg, J. M. Fritsch, J. Vernikos-Danellis. "Head Down Bed Rest Impairs Vagal Baroreflex Responses and Provokes Orthostatic Hypotension." *Journal of Applied Physiology* 68 (1990): 1458-1464.

Cox, J. F., K. U. O. Tahvanainen, T. A. Kuusela, B. D. Levine, W. H. Cooke, T. Mano, S. Iwase, M. Saito, Y. Sugiyama, A. C. Ertl, I. Biaggioni, A. Diedrich, R. M. Robertson, J. H. Zuckerman, L. D. Lane, C. A. Ray, R. J. White, J. A. Pawelczyk, J. C. Buckey,Jr., F. J. Baisch, C. G. Blomquist, D. Robertson, D. L. Eckberg. "Influence of Microgravity on Sympathetic and Vagal Responses to Valsalva's Manoeuver." *Journal of Physiology (London)* 538 (2002): 300-322.

Drummer, C., C. Hesse, F. Baisch, P. Norsk, B. Elmann-Larsen, R. Gerzer, M. Heer. "Water and Sodium Balances and their Relation to Body Mass Changes in Microgravity." *European Journal of Clinical Investigation* 30 (2000):1066-1075.

Ertl, A. C., A. Diedrich, S. Y. Paranjape, I. Biaggioni, R. M. Robertson, L. D. Lane, R. Shiavi, D. Robertson. "The Sympathetic Nervous System Response to Spaceflight." In: *The Neurolab Spacelab Mission: Neuroscience Research in Space,* J.C.Buckey, J.L.Homick, Eds. NASA SP-2003-535, pp197-202, 2003.

Ferrari, A. U., A. Radaeli, M. Cantola. "Aging and the Cardiovascular System." *Journal Applied Physiology* 95 (2003): 2591-2597.

Heer, M., F. Baisch, J. Kropp, R. Gerzer, C. Drummer. "High Dietary Sodium Chloride Consumption may not Induce Body Fluid Retention in Humans." *American Journal of Physiology* 278 (2000): F585-F595.

Rossum, A., M. Ziegler, J. Meck. "Effect of Spaceflight on Cardiovascular Responses to Upright Posture in a 77-year-old Astronaut." *American Journal of Cardiology* 88 (2001): 1335-1337.

Titze, J., M. Shakibaei, M. Schafflhuber. "Glycosaminoglycan Polymerization may Enable Osmotically Inactive Na+ Storage in the Skin." *American Journal of Physiology* (2004, in press).
www.pilates-studio.com for a list of authorized instructors.

Chapter 6

Cacciopo, J. T., L. C. Hawkley, G. G. Bernston, J. M. Ernst, A. C. Gibbs, R. Stickgold, I. A. Hobson. "Lonely Days Invade the Night: Social Modulation of Sleep Efficiency" *Psychological Science* 13 (2002): 385-388.

Czeisler, C. A., J. F. Duffy, T. L. Shanahan, E. N. Brown, J. F. Mitchell, D. W. Rimmer, J. M. Ronda, E. J. Silva, D. T. Emens, D. T. Dijk, R. E. Kronauer. "Stability, Precision, and Near-24-hour Period of the Human Pacemaker." *Science*, 284 (1999):2177-2181.

Dijk, D. J., D. F. Neri, J. K. Wyatt, J. M. Ronda, E. Riel, A. Ritz-De Cecco, R. T. Hughes, A. R. Elliott, G. K. Prisk, J. B. West. "Sleep, Performance, Circadian Rythms, and Light-dark Cycles during Two Space Shuttle Flights." *American Journal of Physiology* 281 (2001): R1647-1664.

Dinges, D. F., F. Pack, K. Williams, K.A. Gillen, T. W. Powell, G. E. Ott, C. Aptowitz, A. I. Pack. "Cumulative Sleepiness, Mood Disturbance and Psychomotor Vigilance Performance Decrements during a Week of Sleep Restricted to 4-5 Hours per Night." *Sleep* 20 (1997): 267-277.

Monk, T. H., S. K. Kennedy, L. R. Rose, J. M. Linenger. "Decreased Human Circadian Pacemaker Influence after 100 Days in Space: A Case Study." *Psychosomatic Medicine* 63 (2001): 881-885.

Natani, K., J. Y. Shurley, C. M. Pierce, R. E. Brooks. "Long Term Changes in Sleep Patterns in Men on the South Polar Plateau" *Archives of Internal Medicine* 125 (1970): 655-659.

Rayl, A. J. S. "Research Turns another 'Fact' into Myth" *The Scientist,* 13 (1999): 16.

Saletu, B., G. M. Saletu-Zyhlarz. *Was Sie Schon Immer über Schlaf Wissen Wollten (Everything You Always Wanted to Know about Sleep)* Vienna: Ueberreuter Verlag, 2002.

Chapter 7

Katz, L. C. *Keep Your Brain Alive*, Workman Publishing, 1999.

Lerner, Alan J. "Alzheimer's Disease in Males: Endocrine Issues and Prospects." *Journal of Clinical Endocrinology and Metabolism* 84 (1999): 3416-3419.

Maki, P. M., S. M. Resnik. "Longitudinal Effects of Estrogen Replacement Therapy on PET Cerebral Blood Flow and Cognition." *Neurobiology of Aging*, 21 (2000): 373-383.

Etnier, J. L., D. M. Landers. "Brain Function and Exercise: Current Perspectives" *Sports Medicine* 19 (1995): 81-85.

Restak, R. M. *Older and Wiser: How to Maintain Peak Mental Ability for as Long as You Live*, New York: Simon and Schuster, 1997.

Schacter, D. L. *Searching for memory: The Brain, the Mind, and the Past*, New York: Basic Books, 1996.

Tanzi, R. E., A. B. Parsons. *Decoding Darkness: The Search for the Genetic Causes of Alzheimer's Disease*. Cambridge: Perseus Books, 2000.

Budzynski, T. H. *Neurobics* Tapes and CDs, Mindbyte Inc., 2001.

DANA Alliance for Brain Initiatives, www.dana.org

National Institute on Mental Health
    www.nimh.nih.gov
    www.brainbuilder.com
    http://snow.utoronyo.ca/learn2/mod4/mnemonics.html

Chapter 8

Cacciopo, J. T., J. M.Ernst, M. H. Burleson, M. K. McClintock, W. B. Malarkey, L. C. Hawkley, R. B. Kowaleski, A. Paulsen, I. A. Hobson, K. Hugdahl, D. Speigel, G. G. Bernston. "Lonely Traits and Concomitant

Physiological Processes: the MacArthur Social Neuroscience Studies." *International Journal of Psychphysiology* 35 (2000): 143-154.

Cannon, W. B. *The Wisdom of the Body.* New York: Norton, 1932.

Chroussos, G. P., P. W. Gold. "The Concepts of Stress and Stress System Disorders." *Journal of the American Medical Association* 267 (1992):1244-1252.

Chroussos, G. P. *The Stress Response and Immune Function: Clinical Implications, The 1999 Novera H. Spector Lecture,* Annals of the New York Academy of Science 917 (2000): 38-67.

Cockburn, A., A. K. Lee. "Marsupial Femme Fatale." *Natural History,* March 1988.

Conner, R. L., J. Vernikos-Danellis, S. Levine, "Stress, Fighting and Neuroendocrine Function." *Nature (London)* 234 (1971):564-566.

Cousins, N. *The Anatomy of an Illness,* New York: Bantam Doubleday Dell, 1991.

Lazarus, R. S. *Psychological Stress and the Coping Process.* New York: McGraw-Hill, 1966.

Li,J., D. H. Precht, P. B. Mortensen, J. Olsen. "Mortality in Parents after Death of a Child in Denmark: a Nationwide Follow-up Study." *The Lancet* 361(2003): 363-367.

Mahoney, D., R. M. Restak. *The Longevity Strategy: How to Live to 100 Using the Brain-Body Connection,* New York: The Dana Press/John Wiley and Sons Inc. 1998.

Rosenman, R. H., R. J. Brand, R. I. Sholtz, M. Friedman. "Multivariate Prediction of Coronary Heart Disease During 8.5 year Follow-up in the Western Collaborative Group Study." *American Journal of Cardiology* 37 (1976): 903.

Seligman, M. E. P. *Helplessness,* San Francisco: W.H.Freeman, 1975.

Selye, H. "A Syndrome Produced by Diverse Nocuous Agents." *Nature (London)* 138 (1936): 32.

Vernikos-Danellis, J., W. L. Goldenrath, C. B. Dolkas. "The Physiological Cost of Flight Stress and Flight Fatigue." *U.S. Navy Medicine*, 66 (1975): 12-16.

Chapter 9

Burton, R. R., A. H. Smith. "Increased Chronic Acceleration Exposure Enhances Work Capacity." *Journal of Gravitational Physiology* 4 (1997): 15-20.

Fiatarone, M. A., E. F. O'Neill, D. Ryan, K. M. Clements, G. R. Solares, M. E. Nelson, S. B. Roberts, J. J. Kehayas, L. A. Lipsitz, W. J. Evans. "Exercise Training and Nutritional Supplementation for Physical Frailty in Very Elderly People." *New England Journal of Medicine* 330 (1974): 1769-1775.

Fuller, P. M., C. H. Warden, S. J. Barry, C. A. Fuller. "Effects of 2G Exposures on Temperature Regulation, Circadian Rhythms and Adiposity in UCP 2/3 Transgenic Mice." *Journal of Applied Physiology* 89 (2000): 1491-1498.

Fuller, P. M., T. A. Jones, S. M. Jones, C. A. Fuller. "Neurovestibular Modulation of Circadian and Homeostatic Regulation: Vestibulohypothalamic Connection?" *Proceedings of the National Academy of Sciences* 99 (2002): 15723-15728.

Lane, H. W., D. A. Schoeller. *Nutrition in Spaceflight and Weightlessness Models*, Boca Raton: CRC Press LLC, 2000.

Nestle, M. *Food Politics*, San Francisco: California University Press. 2002.

Perricone, N. *The Perricone Prescription*. New York: Harper Collins Publishers, Inc. 2002.

Seddon, M. R., M. J. Fettman, R. W. Phillips. "Practical and Clinical Nutritional Concerns during Space Flight." *American Journal of Nutrition* 60 (1994):825S-830S.

Sen, C. K., L. Packer, O. Hanninen, (Eds.) *Exercise and Oxygen Toxicity*. NewYork: Elsevier, 1994.

Smith, A. H. "Effects of Chronic Acceleration in Animals." *Life Sciences and space Research* 11 (19): 201-206.

Somer, E. *The Origin Diet*, New York: Henry Holt and Company, 2001. www.mendosa.com/gi.htm

Chapter 10

Finch, C. E. *Longevity, Senescence, and the Genome*. Chicago: University of Chicago Press, 1990.

Jazwinski, S. M. "Longevity, Genes and Aging" Science, 273 (1996): 54-59.

Lithgow, G. J., T. B. L. Kirkwood. "Mechanism and Evolution of Aging" *Science*, 273 (1996): 80.

Pearl, R. *The Rate of Living*, New York: Knopf, 1928.

Walford, R.L. *Maximum Life Span*, New York: W.W.Norton, 1983.

Warshofsky, F. *"Stealing Time: The New Science of Aging"* New York: TV Books, 1999.

Weindruch, R. "Caloric Restriction and Aging," *Scientific American*, 274 (1996): 46-52.

Chapter 11

Butler, R. N. *"Why Survive? Being Old in America,"* New York: Harper & Row, 1975.

Butler, R. N. *"Love and Sex after Forty,"* New York: Harper Collins Publishers, 1990.

Clement, G., A. Pavy-Le Traon. "Centrifugation as a Countermeasure during Actual and Simulated Microgravity: A Review." *European Journal of Applied Physiology* 92 (2004): 235-248.

Murakami, D. M., L. Erkman, O. Hermanson, M. G. Rosenfeld, A. C. Fuller. "Evidence of Vestibular Regulation of Autonomic Functions in a Mouse Genetic Model." *Proceedings of the National Academy of Sciences* 99 (2002):17078-17082.

Perls, T. T. "The Oldest Old." *Scientific American*, 272 (1995): 70-75.

Peterson, P. G. "Gray Dawn: The Global Aging Crisis." *Foreign Affairs* 78 (1999): 42-55.

Peterson, P. G. *Gray Dawn: How the Coming Age Wave will Transform America—and the World.* New York: Times Book, 1999.

Roszak, T. *America the Wise*, New York: Houghton Mifflin Company, 1998.

Rowe, J. W., R. L. Kahn. *Successful Aging: The MacArthur Foundation Study. New York:* Dell Trade Publishing, 1998.

Vernikos, J., D. A. Ludwig, A. C. Ertl, C. E. Wade, L. C. Keil, D. O'Hara. "Effect of Standing or Walking on Physiological Changes Induced by Head Down Bed Rest." *Aviation, Space and Environmental Medicine* 67 (1996):1069-1079.

Vernikos, J. "Artificial Gravity: Intermittent Centrifugation as a Spaceflight Countermeasure." *Journal of Gravitational Physiology* 4 (1997): P13-16.

World Demographic Trends, Report of the Secretary General, E/cN.9/1995/5, United Nations Economic and Social Council, Commission on Population and Development.

National Center for Health Statistics (NCHS)
 Centers for Disease Control and Prevention
 3311 Toledo Road
 Hyattsville, MD 20782
 Email: nchsquery@cdc.gov
 Website: www.cdc.gov/nchs

Acknowledgements

One does not realize just how many different groups of people and talents are involved in putting together a book of this nature. My research colleagues and friends Gig Levine, Mary Dallman, Vic Convertino, Jack Barchas, Glenn Van Loon, Lanny Keil, Hal Sandler, and Carolyn Leach Huntoon worked with me on the bed-rest studies and collaborated for no financial gain (unheard of in NASA). Dee O'Hara ensured the studies were done right.

The many very special men and women who volunteered to lie in bed and be poked and tested, some more than once, must have wondered whether the research would ever bear fruit. Bob Norby, Ron Sopp, Will Golden, Joe Dimers, Sam, Russ Nelson, Ross Ross, Bill McClain, Bob Bowers, Glenn Stover, Kay Holley, Linda Willis, Karen Kettlety, Nancy Muchia and her risqué jokes, Carol Yanz, Lynn Hines, Consuelo Bennett, Candace Eng, Judy Demers, Ann Hutchison...and all the others, this is for you.

Equally, I want to thank the many active seniors at my tennis club as well as friends, neighbors, parents of friends, relatives, emeritus scientists, and people I stopped in supermarkets and even in the street who willingly shared their secrets to staying young and active. My uncle Nicolas, who did not quite reach his one hundredth birthday this year, practiced what I preach. My very special friend Gus Matthews listened and argued as I worked my way through many theories. My walking partner Judy Buzzell was the target of my lectures as were the rest of the Bon Appetit Sisterhood who were an inspiration throughout. They will be gorgeous and dynamic when they turn 100!

Richard Hodes, director, and Fox Wetle, his deputy, at the National Institute on Aging gave me positive feedback as we shared the interesting times surrounding Senator Glenn's return into space. I benefited from our constructive discussions, as I did from those with Meredith Hay at the University of Missouri.

This list would not be complete without naming the indomitable Tom Rogers, who over many years reinforced my belief in the importance of bringing to the fore the special role space played in our understanding of aging. Thanks to Bob Butler, the first to point out that aging is not a disease. Interviews with AARP, the President's Council on Physical Fitness, and other organizations concerned with aging helped me refine this theory.

Special thanks to Emily Holton, David Tomko, Chrys Papadeli, and Greg and Pamela Copley, who reviewed parts of the text as it evolved. I am deeply grateful to Ralph Pelligra, Dee O'Hara, Harry Guy, Charles Billings, and the Hon. Hans Mark, who went over the entire manuscript with a fine-tooth comb and provided me with invaluable constructive advice that greatly improved the end product.

I could not have done this book without the heroic help of our very dear friend Robin Hosie, co-writer and editor, who worked so hard and with great tact to turn my writing into plain English. Barbara Marshall, my agent, was quick to see the compelling nature of the subject and the challenge I presented. Her patience, advice, and professional guidance have been invaluable.

Special thanks to those who believed in me: Hind Sadek, Don Hilty, Mary Anne Frey and most of all my very special Geoffrey, who never allowed me to give up. It has been another great adventure.

Joan Vernikos
August 2004

0-595-32931-4

Made in the USA
Lexington, KY
28 August 2014